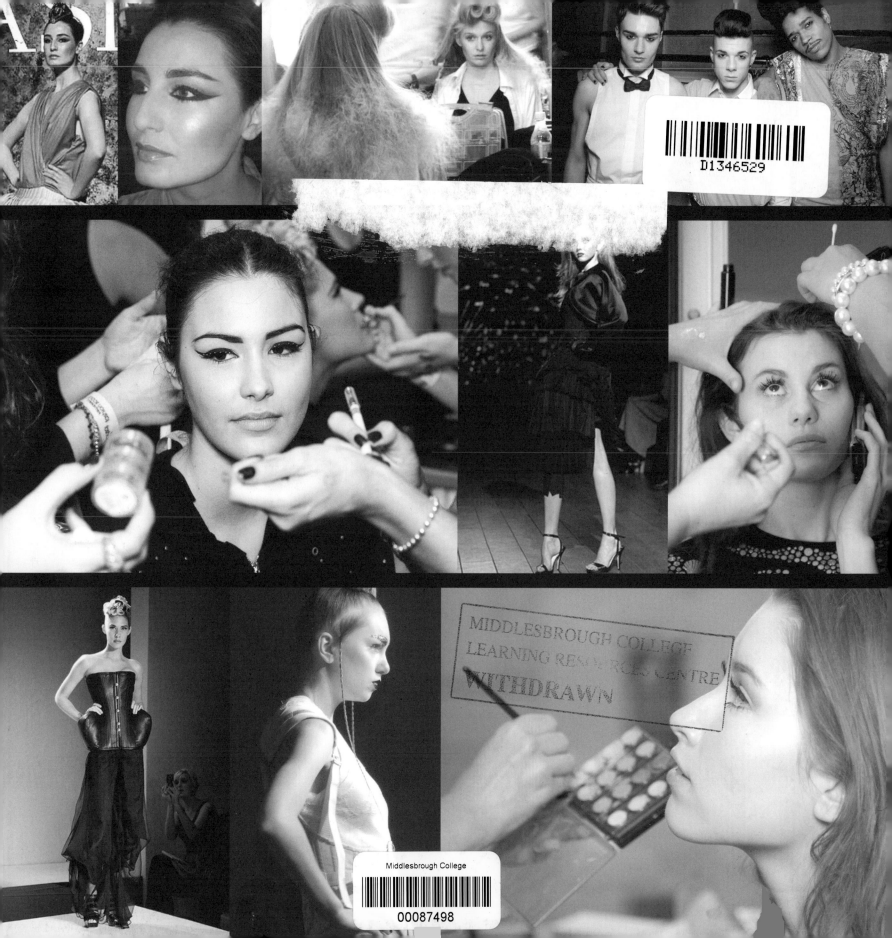

MAKEUP IS ART

Professional techniques for creating original looks

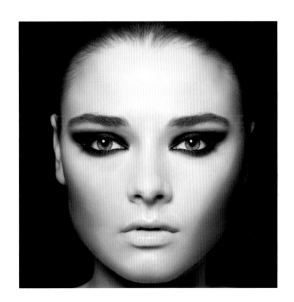

"Dedicated to my loving Grandmother Mavis Kenneally.
Without you this would have not been possible."

JANA

This edition published in 2010
by Carlton Books Limited
20 Mortimer Street
London W1T 3JW

10 9 8 7 6 5 4 3 2 1

Printed and bound in China

Creative Directors: Jana Ririnui and Lan Nguyen

Copyeditors: Sarah-Jane Corfield-Smith and Jane Donovan

Makeup artists: Lan Nguyen, Jana Ririnui, Sandra Cooke, Rachel Wood, Jose Bass, Jo
Sugar, Lina Dahlbeck, Philippe Milleto, Christina Iravedra, Carolyn Roper, Jade Hunka,
Nat Van Zee, Maria Papaodpoulou, Elsebeth Tan, Sharka P.

Contributing writers: Lan Nguyen, Jana Ririnui, Sandra Cooke, Rachel Wood, Jo Sugar,
Barbra Villasenor, Lina Dahlbeck, Jose Bass, Sarah-Jane Corfield-Smith, Yvonne Chung,
Carolyn Roper.

Photographers: Camille Sanson, Catherine Harbour, Fabrice Lachant, Keith Clouston,
Jason Ell, Desmond Murray, Conrad Atton, Zoe Barling, Mo Saito, Han Lee de Boer,
Allan Chiu, Roberto Aguliar, Daniel Nadel, Lou Denim, Dez Mighty.

Hair Stylists: Jana Ririnui, Marc Eastlake, Desmond Murray, Zoe Irwin, Andrea Cassolari,
Nathalie Malbert, Natasha Mygdal, Cyndia Harvey, Fabio Vivan, Tim Furssedonn,
Zach Jardin.

Stylists: Rebekah Roy, Karl Willett, Shyla Hassan, Nasrin Jean-Batiste, Svetlana Prodanic,
David Hawkins, Sampson Soboye, Zed-Eye.

Front cover Photography by Camille Sanson, makeup by Lan Nguyen, head piece by
Mrac Eastlake Design using Swarovski. **Overleaf** Photography by Lou Denim, makeup
by Jade Hunka using MAC, model Jodie @ Nevs.

Original book design by Disciple Productions.

MAKEUP IS ART

Professional techniques for creating original looks

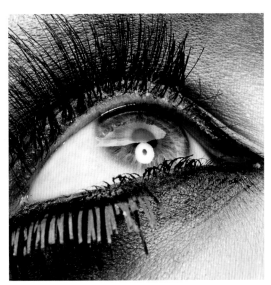 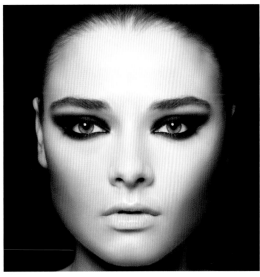 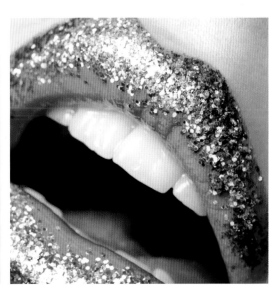

JANA RIRINUI & LAN NGUYEN

CARLTON
BOOKS

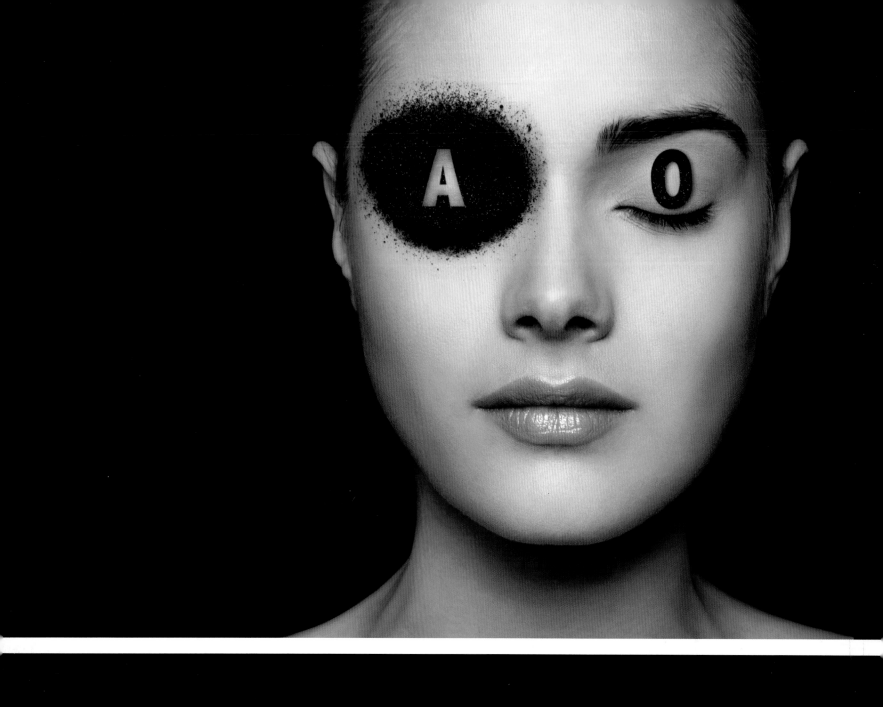

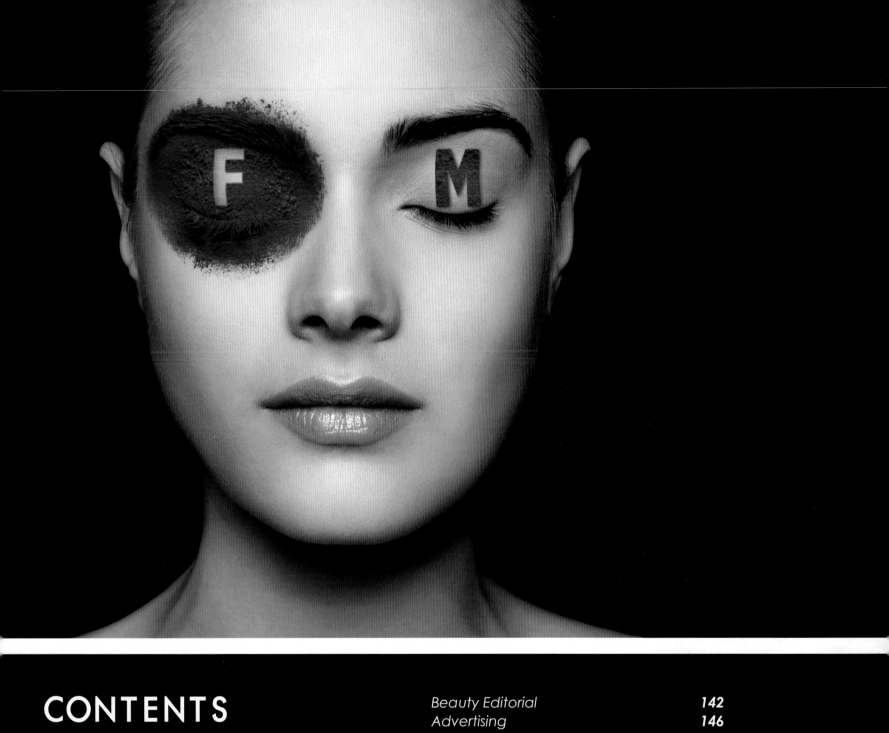

CONTENTS

JANA RIRINUI

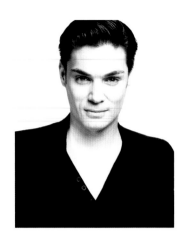

Jana Ririnui, Makeup Artist and Founder of AOFM

"I was born in New Zealand in a small town called Invercargill, far away from the fast pace of a fashion capital like London. I started my career at 14, working for free at a hair salon after school. My dream was to become a hairdresser and I was prepared to work hard to make this a reality. I moved to Australia where there were more opportunities, allowing me to build up my hairdressing skills. It was here that I was spotted and approached by a modelling agency and started to model. Although it took me away from my hairdressing, modelling gave me a wider perspective of the fashion world and experience on the other side of the camera. It was here that I realized that makeup artistry is where my heart belonged. I decided to move to London in 1999, knowing it would be the perfect place to combine my skills as a hairdresser with my potential as a makeup artist.

I studied at one of London's well-known schools, but upon completion of my courses as a makeup student, I felt a little lost as no-one had really prepared me for the hard road ahead or how competitive the industry was going to be. Despite the lack of guidance I worked really hard on my career and after painstaking work and testing with photographers I eventually found my feet as a makeup artist. Looking back. I took every opportunity to work – as long as I was applying makeup, I was happy. I worked on cosmetic counters, shooting on my days off with photographers and assisting for free just to gain more experience. I do not think I really began to learn about the industry until I started assisting other makeup artists. This all helped lead me to become a successful artist. I have worked on a number of famous magazines along with some big names, but my passion has always been the desire to teach and provide help to aspiring makeup artists who were in the same situation as me when I finished my training.

While talking to friends and fellow makeup artists about setting up a school, it was felt there was a need to offer training conducted by professional, working makeup artists. As the industry is so small and competitive it seemed clear to us that the best people to teach makeup skills and industry know-how are those who are already successful artists themselves. I didn't get to learn about the industry until I was undertaking jobs, so I wanted to ensure my students would have the opportunity to understand the workings of the profession whilst developing their skills.

So the Academy was born – the first in the industry to be owned and operated by freelance makeup artists with a love of the industry. My desire is to encourage the next generation of makeup artists, giving them the tools, knowledge and understanding that is essential to succeed. My philosophy has seen AOFM's reputation grow as one of the leading makeup schools and our students have gone on to become some of the finest and most successful international freelance makeup artists, as well as top fashion and beauty editors for major magazines and newspapers.

I formed the AOFM Pro team, which has become a well-known creative force within the industry, driven by the team's flair and conceptual ideas. We have come together with other top industry professionals to create a book dedicated to inspire other makeup artists, people wishing to enter this exciting career and anyone who appreciates fine art and beauty.

This book is packed full of creative ideas, inside knowledge from our artists' experiences and advice on how this forever-changing industry operates. It will keep you one step ahead of the competition and give you a true insight into the creative world of makeup artistry."

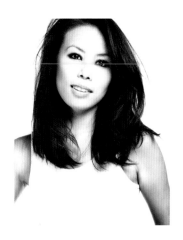

LAN NGUYEN

Lan Nguyen, Makeup Artist and Creative Director

"MAKEUP is ART. This is the true definition of how I see makeup. Every face is a blank canvas and every brushstroke creates something magical. Applying makeup is an art form in itself, but the finished piece is what excites me. My inspiration comes from past and present art, from people and colours and the cosmetic products available around me. I love makeup and consider it a very important tool to help not only enhance your own natural beauty, but to build confidence for everyday life. When you feel good, you look good, and makeup helps you achieve this positive feeling.

Painting has always been a part of my life. From an early age it was all I did – poster competitions, portraits, landscape watercolour paintings. Even though I was advised to do something more mainstream as a career I refused and followed my heart, which was art, where I knew at least I would be happy. I used every art medium available at the time and just wanted to create, whether it was on canvas, paper, clothes, walls or doors! Every blank space was my canvas.

I studied art and fashion design at Central Saint Martins College of Art and Design, and it was here that I began my journey into the fashion industry. At college, I learned the disciplines of concept, design, creating and working with materials around me, which has been a philosophy I still apply to my work as a makeup artist today. It was during this time that I discovered that working as a makeup artist could be a successful profession.

While working as a runner at a photography studio, I was handed a set of makeup brushes and asked to help out on a busy shoot, which turned out to be not only a success, but a major turning point my life. With no experience in the makeup field, I simply treated my model like a painting and did what I thought was best.

Working and learning on the job was my form of training and I took every opportunity to experiment and develop my skills as a professional makeup artist. I networked with other makeup artists, stylists and photographers and this led me to my first collaboration on a professional high-fashion test shoot for my portfolio.

Afterwards, I was invited to assist a fashion and news photographer whom I'd met by chance. This chance meeting took me to New York, London, Milan and Paris fashion weeks. The whole experience inspired me to embrace the business of becoming a makeup artist seriously.

Seeing it all happen before my eyes was an amazing process, and gave me the drive and realization that this was what I wanted to do. I questioned some of the top makeup artists at the shows who gave me sound advice.

I had gained invaluable knowledge by working backstage, interviewing models and dealing with picture editors from around the world and by simply being steeped in the whole process and industry. Words cannot describe the magic that happens when everyone is working under pressure as a team to produce a beautiful show.

As a makeup artist, I am always learning on the job. I get given a lot of freedom, which allows me to develop different techniques and create what I like. Some of my ideas are accidental, which have then developed into exciting projects. There is so much creativity around us and by producing this book I have only touched on one of many visions.

It has been a great pleasure collaborating with my fellow models, makeup artists, hair stylists, fashion stylists, designers, photographers and agents, especially the Academy of Freelance Makeup. Without their support I would not have been able to achieve what I have accomplished so far. For this I would like to say a personal thank you to all."

SKINCARE

As a makeup artist, it helps to understand skin, as it is the canvas that you work on. If you prepare and look after the skin well, then your makeup will sit better and last longer. It is fully recommended to study the skin to the level of a beautician, as this will help you understand makeup application more fully.

It is not necessary to carry a skincare range for each skin type in your makeup kit. However, it is important to be able to manage and control each skin type to your advantage. Many tutors at AOFM and makeup artists are big fans of Dermalogica. It is a brand that acknowledges the importance of skin and creates products that make the makeup artist's job easier, as well as offers ongoing training for makeup artists lucky enough to be included on their artist list. The following pages will guide you through the essential skincare products for an artist's kit.

When choosing a skincare range, opt for one that is not highly perfumed and is suitable for use on sensitive skin. Models have makeup applied and removed so frequently that their skin becomes easily sensitized. It is also important to carry a good-quality range if you plan to work with celebrities – which is why, for so many makeup artists, Dermalogica ticks the boxes.

When doing pre-recorded television, videos, bridal makeup, beauty and fashion shoots, and celebrity makeup, always use a full range of products, including cleanser, toner and moisturizer, unless the celebrity requests their own preferred brand and products. Live television or shooting on location often requires wipes and moisturizer to save time. On fashion shows, if time allows, use a full range, but when pushed for time it is essential to carry wipes.

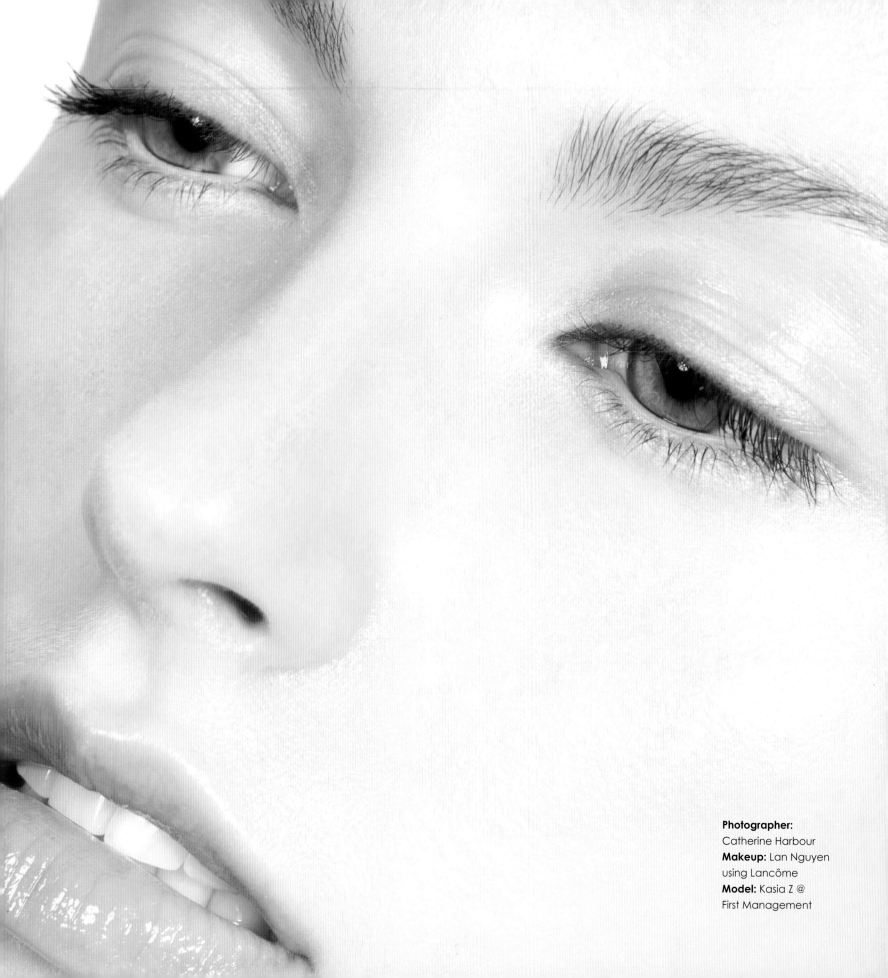

Photographer:
Catherine Harbour
Makeup: Lan Nguyen
using Lancôme
Model: Kasia Z @
First Management

PRODUCTS & PREPARATION

It is important to pay attention to dry and oily skin. Dry skin needs oil and moisture put back into it, so skin preparation and products containing oil and moisture will help the makeup last longer. If you do not treat dry skin you may experience flaking, which will ruin your foundation. Oily skin needs products that help reduce shine and oil. Skincare and makeup products containing oil will cause your makeup to slide, and shine will be visible very quickly, making the makeup difficult to manage.

Cleansers
An ultra-calming cream cleanser is an effective and gentle cleanser that is mild enough to be used to remove eye makeup. Is also convenient on location as it can be removed without water. Face wipes, such as MAC and Simple, can be used instead of cleanser and toner for speed and convenience. These are commonly used backstage and on photo shoots to remove makeup quickly and efficiently.

Toners
Use a convenient spray toner that is gentle, moisturizing and refreshing. It helps prepare the skin for moisturizer, and does not need to be removed.

Treatments for Eyes and Lips
A firming vitamin-packed treatment that contains silicone, which acts like a primer, will smooth wrinkles and moisturize the sensitive skin around the eyes and lips. Lucas Pawpaw Ointment is great to use on dry, chapped lips.

Treating the Problem (optional)
Some skins may require additional treatment for problem areas. For dry skin or to add moisture use a hydrating booster before moisturizing. This can also be used on the lips. For sensitive skin use a gentle treatment for reducing redness and calming the skin. For mature skin or premature ageing, a firming booster or serum can help reduce the appearance of fine lines and wrinkles. For skin prone to breakouts and spots, a clearing spot treatment is effective to help reduce breakouts. Dermalogica has pre-moisturizer boosters for all these conditions.

Moisturizers
Choose your moisturizer according to your skin type. For chronically dry skin, choose a rich, concentrated moisturizer. For normal to dry skin, a medium-weight moisturizer such as Dermalogica's Skin Smoothing Cream is ideal to hydrate and smooth the skin. For oily skin, you will need a light-hydration formula that reduces the appearance of oil and helps close the pores.

Tinted Moisturizers
A tinted moisturizer is used to moisturize the skin as well as provide sheer coverage to help even out skin tone. It is ideal for people that do not want to wear a foundation, but still want a little coverage.

Beauty Serums
Serums are used as part of a facial treatment. Similar to a moisturizer, a serum is a liquid for treating skin conditions such as dehydration, redness, discoloration and fine lines. They contain highly concentrated ingredients that are absorbed into the skin quickly and more deeply for an intensive effect. The high concentration of skin-benefiting ingredients penetrates into the skin, producing dramatic and long-lasting results.

To use, apply a drop of serum to your fingertips and massage it gently into skin in the morning and at night, then follow with your usual moisturizer. You do not need to use more than a drop or two to cover the whole face and neck. You will probably feel an immediate change in your skin the first time you use a serum – it may feel softer, smoother and perhaps even a little tighter.

Exfoliants

The skin is always generating new skin cells at the lower layer and sending them to the surface. As the cells rise to the surface they gradually die and become filled with keratin. These keratinized skin cells are important because they protect the skin during the creation of new skin cells. As we age, however, the process of cell turnover slows down. Cells start to pile up unevenly on the skin's surface, giving it a dry, rough, dull appearance. Exfoliation is beneficial because it removes the older cells and reveals the fresher, younger skin cells below. It also makes expensive facial products like serums easier to penetrate into the skin.

Only use products designed for the face, as some of those designed for the body can be too abrasive and irritating for the face. A fine powder exfoliant that becomes a paste when mixed with water will smooth out dry, flaky skin and remove dead skin cells. The best method is to use exfoliating gloves or a synthetic scrubbing sponge designed for the face. To do this, gently rub your face with the sponge using circular motions. Avoid scrubbing under the eyes, where the skin is thin and can easily be damaged. The residue can be removed with warm water or damp cotton wool pads.

Exfoliating can cause the skin to dry out, and dry skin is an invitation for skin to wrinkle. By over-exfoliating you run the risk of bursting the delicate blood vessels under the skin as well, and if the vessels burst, your skin may appear permanently flushed.

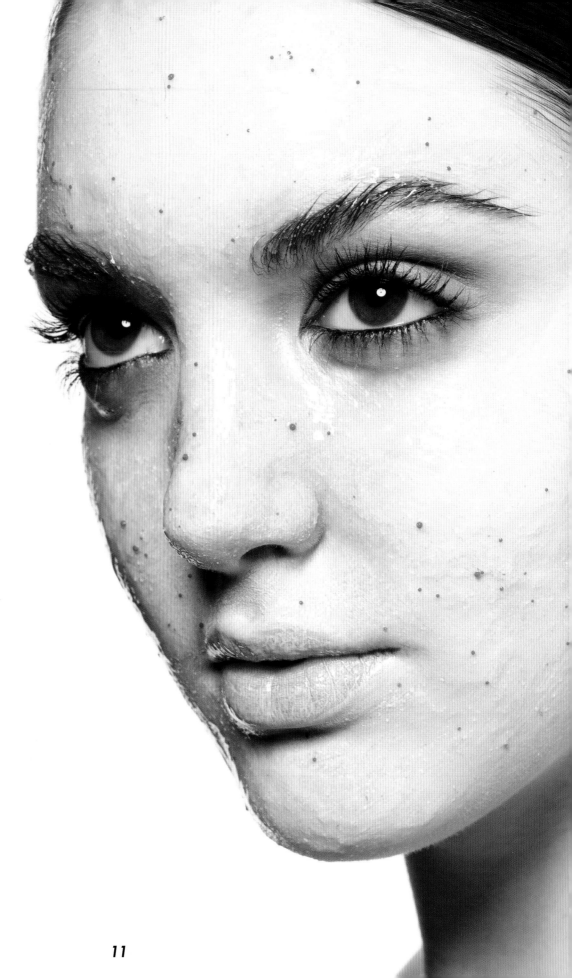

Photographer:
Catherine Harbour
Makeup: Lan Nguyen
using Lancôme **Model:**
Rosanne F @ Premier

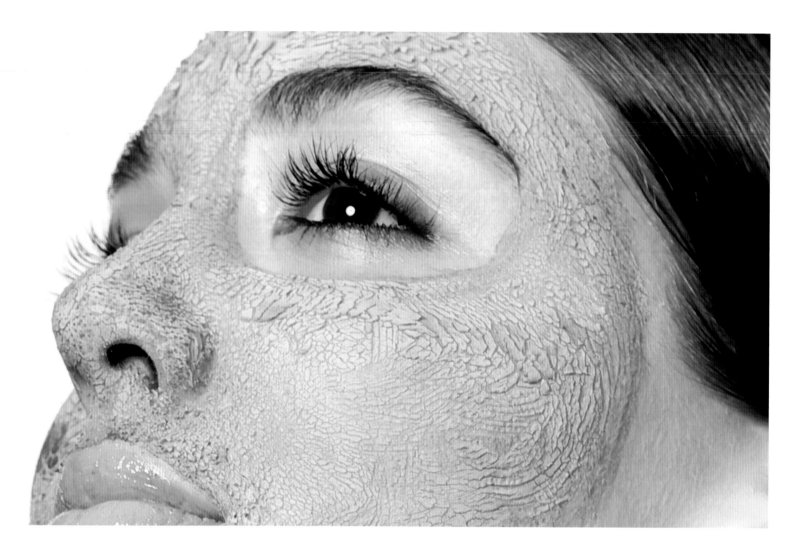

Face Masks

Masks can make the difference between good skin and great skin. There is a different one appropriate for every skin type. Facial masks will exfoliate your skin and remove any buildup of sluggish cells. A face mask, along with daily skin washes, will keep your pores unclogged and help clear up blemishes by stimulating blood circulation. When the seasons change your skin also changes, so you may need to switch your mask with the change in weather. Most are best applied once or twice weekly.

Clay Masks

Best for those with oily skin, clay masks draw out toxins and impurities and are essential for keeping the skin clear.

Peel-off Masks

Intended for the gentle removal of dead skin cells, peel-off masks leave your complexion replenished and radiant. They work with all skin types.

Paraffin Masks

For hydrating and softening the skin, paraffin wax masks are appropriate for all skin types. They aid blood circulation, which will brighten the complexion.

Pore Strips

For the instant removal of blackheads, oil and dirt, and to minimize pores, use pore strips. They have twice the effectiveness of pore-cleansing facial washes and are handy to have in your kit to prevent clogged pores and breakouts. You achieve instant results and the strips can be used up to three times a week.

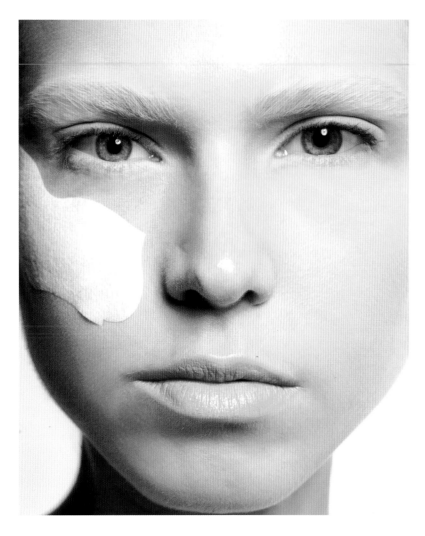

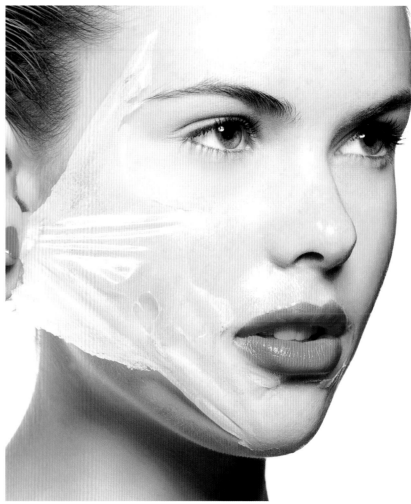

Applying a Mask

Try to use a facial mask at least three times a month. Applying a mask requires a specific technique, but most of us do not know that – we just plaster it all over the place. The first step is to use a flat, wide brush or spatula. Avoid using your fingers!

1 Start applying the mask with a brush or spatula from the centre of face outward, using even strokes. Be careful to avoid the lips and the sensitive area around the eyes.

2 Leave the mask on for at least 20 minutes, unless a particular time frame is mentioned on the packaging. Never leave your mask on the skin for more time than recommended by the manufacturer. Some ingredients could harm the skin if they stay on for longer than necessary.

3 To remove the mask, moisten with a little water and gently rub it off the skin, working one area at a time. In the case of peel-off masks, you will have to peel! Finish by rinsing the face with plenty of water, using circular strokes to remove any residue.

Photographer:
Catherine Harbour
Makeup: Lan Nguyen
and Jade Hunka using
Lancôme **Models:**
Kathleen B (left) and
Gabriele D (right)
@ Premier

THE FACE

In today's society, how you look matters. When creating the perfect look for your client, skin, makeup, hair and nails are all areas that need attention. It is important for an artist to be able to cover skills in these areas confidently, even if there are specialists available. It also helps keep the job diverse and interesting.

Cosmetic products are constantly changing. New products become available and existing ones are improved. It is important to know the ingredients and to be guided by the specialist suppliers. It is also beneficial to test the products first in case a model has become sensitive or allergic. Ultimately it will save you time and avoid costly mistakes.

The freedom of style, that is so prevalent now, allows us to experiment by mixing the classic with the new, and by adding your own signature twist to gives it an edge. Trends always get repeated but as products change they can produce a completely different look.

There are so many timeless beauty icons to use as inspiration but the important rule is that you enhance the facial features to make the model look beautiful. For example, by having a flawless base and then just a touch of colour you can create something that is fun and strong but still gives a beautiful effect.

Photographer:
Jason Ell **Makeup:**
Jose Base using Shu
Uemura **Hair:** Natasha
Mygdal using Bumble
& Bumble **Model:**
Hannah @ Next

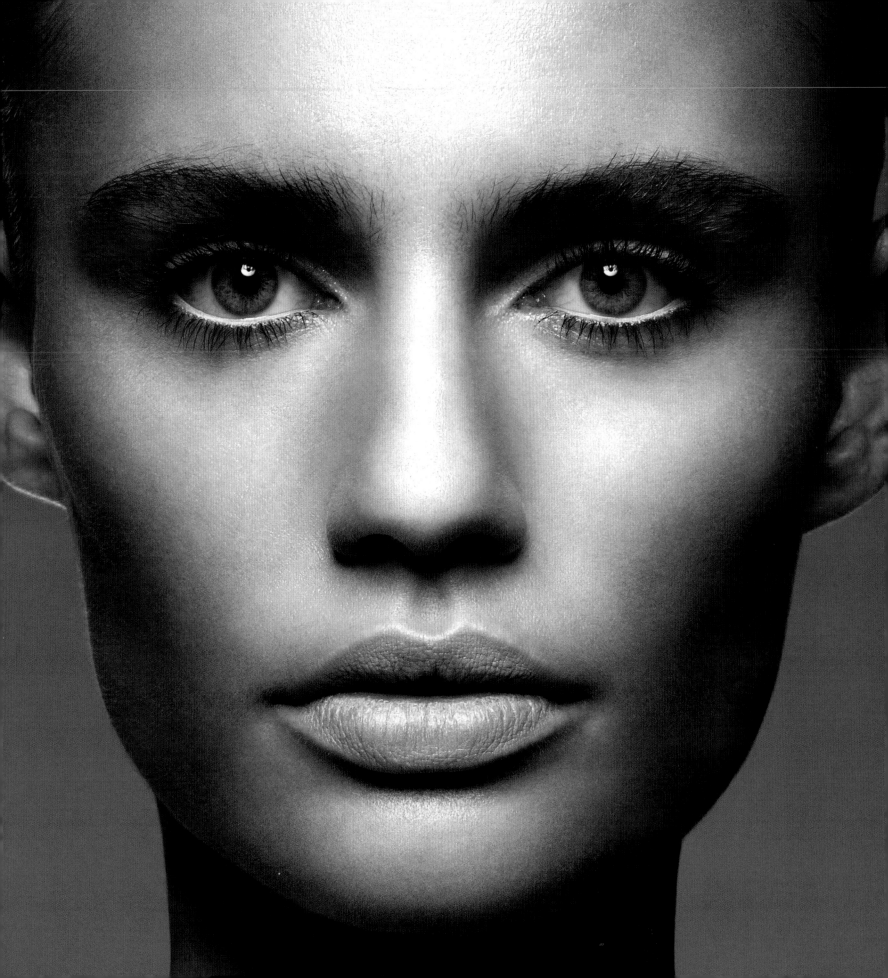

FACE SHAPES

The oval face shape is no longer considered the ideal "perfect" face shape. With today's cultural diversity, we embrace the beauty within everyone. As much as it is useful to know your face shape, it no longer determines what makeup suits you. Instead, use your face shape as a guide to maximizing your natural beauty. Along with cosmetics, your hair style will also help accentuate your face shape.

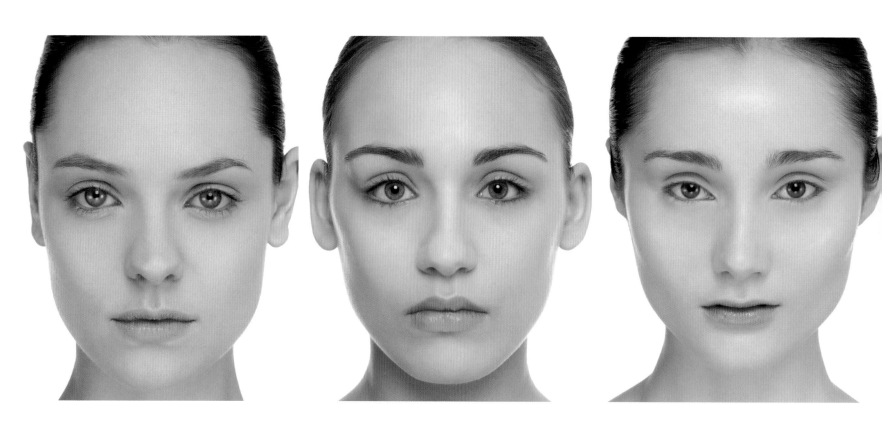

Oval
Once considered the ideal face shape because of its perfect proportions and symmetry, the oval face is generally slightly broader at the cheeks and narrower at the forehead and chin. Little (if any) contouring is needed as the face is well balanced. A good makeup tip is to accentuate your best features. A celebrity example is Kylie Minogue.

Round
This shape face is usually wider than an oval face, with fuller cheeks and often a rounded or non-prominent chin. Round faces tend to have that "baby-face" look. Contour under the cheekbones, on the temples and under the jawline to give the illusion of a more defined bone structure. A celebrity example is Cameron Diaz.

Heart/Inverted Triangle
Wider at the forehead , the heart shape curves to a narrow, pointed chin. For those with an exaggerated heart, the hairline mimics the rounded two bumps of the heart. As it is difficult to soften the prominent chin, accentuate your best feature, such as the eyes or cheeks, to draw attention away from the chin. A celebrity example is Reese Witherspoon.

Photographers:
Keith Clouston and
Catherine Harbour
Makeup: Jade Hunka,
Jo Sugar and Lan
Nguyen using Bobbi
Brown **Models:** Melinte,
Natalie, Elena @
Oxygen, Rosanne F,
Larissa H, Gabriele D
@ Premier

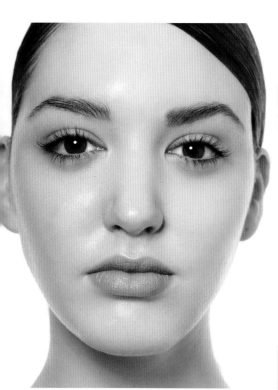 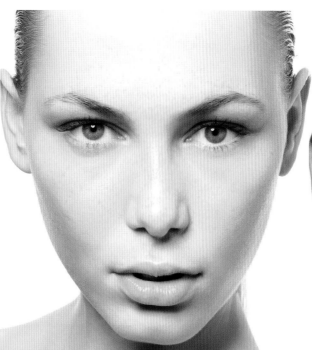 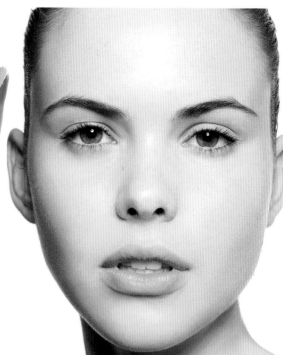

Square

Square faces tend to be a similar width between the forehead, the cheeks and the jawline. Soften square features by contouring under the cheekbones and temples. A celebrity example is Demi Moore.

Triangle

This face type is characterized by a dominant jawline that narrows at the cheekbones and forehead. Contouring under the cheekbones will help add some width to the face. A celebrity example is Victoria Beckham.

Diamond

The forehead and chin are narrower, with wide and inevitably high cheekbones. Little or no contouring is required, simply play up the best features. A celebrity example is Scarlett Johansson.

PRIMERS

A primer is a product that is used to prepare the skin before foundation. For the most part they are all silicon based. The silicon in the product is used to fill in pores and fine lines, to create a smooth base for the foundation or other makeup to be applied. The main benefit of using a primer is that it helps the makeup last longer on the skin.

There are many types of primers available, in the same way that there are numerous moisturizers for different skin types. Primers work best on cleansed, prepared skin, and, if the skin is exceptionally dry, then a primer can be used on the skin after moisturizer.

Types of primers include hydrating ones used for moisturizing dry skin, mattifying for oily skin to help control shine, and primers to plump the skin for a more youthful appearance. Many also contain SPF. Primers can come in a range of textures, such as lotions, mousse, silicon gels, as well as mineral powder primers, specially suited for sensitive skin.

Professional makeup artists, particularly those in the fashion industry, tend to have a range of primers in their kits for use on different jobs. Although in the fashion industry we generally look after models with young, plump skin, and are able to be on set to do touch-ups in between shots, there are still occasions when primers are needed, such as shooting an outdoor editorial where a primer with SPF is essential. Models with tired or dehydrated skin (we see this a lot during fashion week) may require a hydrating primer to help sooth and smooth the skin.

Primers are popular in the television and film industry, where a range of different aged actors and presenters are used. In addition, being on set or on location and under warm lights for long periods of time requires makeup to last longer in between touch-ups.

With the growing industry of high-definition television and film, the amount of makeup worn by actors and presenters needs to be more natural, and yet still effective. As powders can look heavy on television and film, mattifying primers are ideal to help prevent shine and reduce the need for excess powder and continual touch-ups. In addition, on more mature actors and presenters, a silicon-based primer, such as Prep +Prime Skin produced by MAC, will help smooth over fine lines to form a smooth base for foundation to go more flawlessly on to skin. The Becca Line and Pore Corrector is a skin-tone, oil-free primer that can help minimize the pores and lines around the eyes and nose for a smoother base application.

Photographer:
Keith Clouston
Hair and Makeup:
Jana Ririnui using
Becca **Model:**
Yu @ Oxygen

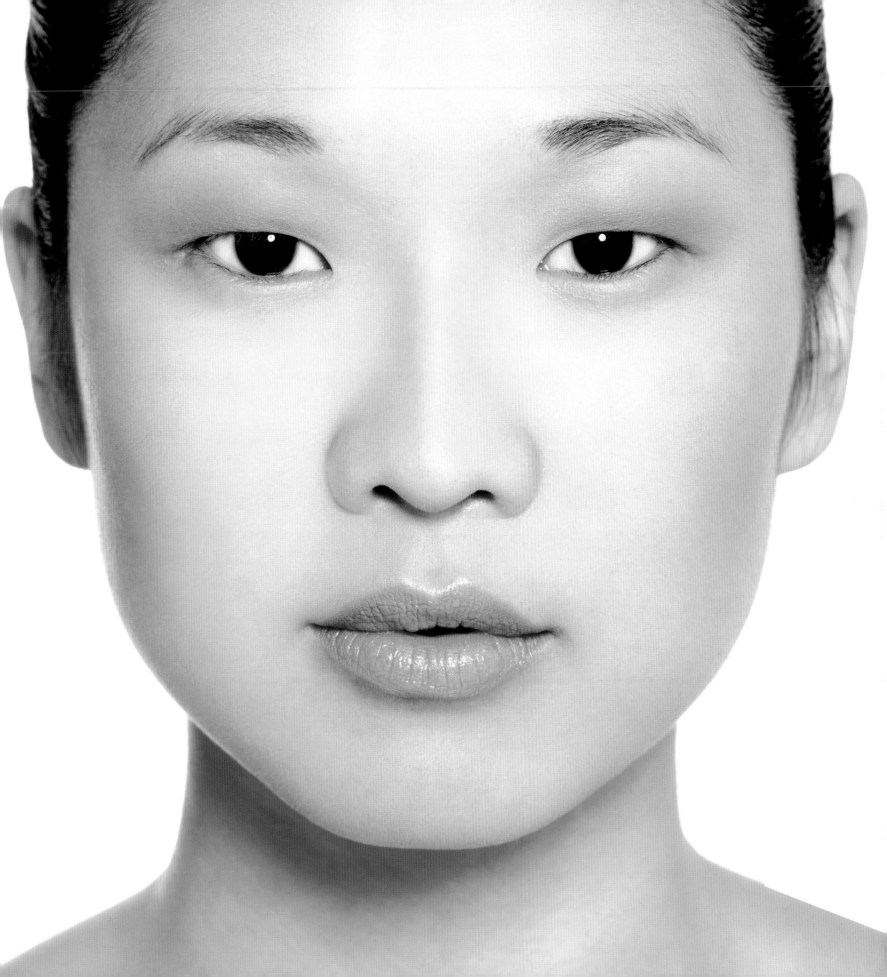

Foundations

The main point of using a foundation or base is to even out the tone and colour of the skin. How a makeup artist wants the skin to appear varies from job to job – all creative briefs differ. On one project a makeup artist may want the skin to have a glow, while on other jobs, an old-fashioned matte, full-coverage base may be needed or the makeup artist may be required to create a natural-looking finish, as if there is no foundation applied at all.

Choosing what type of product to use is one of the biggest challenges a new makeup artist can face. Here is a guide to help sort out the confusion.

Full Coverage

This type of foundation gives skin the appearance of flawlessness. A good full coverage can effectively cover scars, discoloration and blemishes – almost like a concealer – over the entire face. These foundations also work well on Asian and black skin tones.

• To get a flawless base on any skin type, dilute the full coverage or stick foundation by mixing it with a sheer fluid tinted moisturizer.

Sheer Coverage

Sheer foundation lets the skin look natural and unmade. It will even out skin tone, but allows freckles, beauty marks, and so on, to be visible, giving the effect of a makeup-free face.

Oil Free/Oil Control

Great for those with oily skin, this formula can help keep shine at bay by creating a matte-textured finish. Usually "oil free" means it contains no lanolin or mineral oils (these are the oils that tend to clog pores and cause sensitivity).

Illuminating

This is a foundation that leaves a glow and luminous finish on the skin. Some illuminating foundations can contain tiny pearl and glitter particles. When working on photo shoots, it can make the skin look greasy.

Moisturizing

The best base for dry to normal skin types, it gives extra hydration and works well on mature skin.

Cream to Powder

This formula has a more traditional texture and usually comes in a compact. It goes on creamy and dries to a powder finish. Cream-to-powder formulas give a medium finish, which is ideal for skin that needs more coverage than a liquid foundation, but not as much as full coverage.

Powder Based

Best used on oily skin, as it has no liquid or moisture in it, powder-based foundation gives a matte, nonreflective finish to the skin. Another advantage is that it can be used with a brush to set makeup.

Mousse

A whipped product that gives light coverage and a natural glow or matte finish, mousse foundations feel light on the skin.

Tinted Moisturizer

A combination of a moisturizer and some colour, the tinted moisturizer is perfect for evening out the skin tone. It gives a very light coverage and sinks easily into the skin.

• Try using tinted moisturizers if your complexion is dewy, and you are really looking for a light, sheer wash to even out any blotchiness.

Concealers

Used to cover blemishes and imperfections once a foundation has been applied, concealers offer heavier coverage than foundations and also help to cover dark circles under the eyes. When choosing a concealer, you should consider both consistency and colour. It should be lightweight and creamy. The product needs to glide on smoothly and not require a lot of rubbing. Find the right shade and blend it in so it looks flawless, not obvious – it should match your skin exactly. Concealer looks most natural when you work in sheer layers and build it up gradually.

If you are covering major undereye circles, you are going to want a formula that provides heavier coverage. If your skin is sensitive then you should choose a formula that contains only pure mineral pigment colour and no dyes, oils, talc or starch.

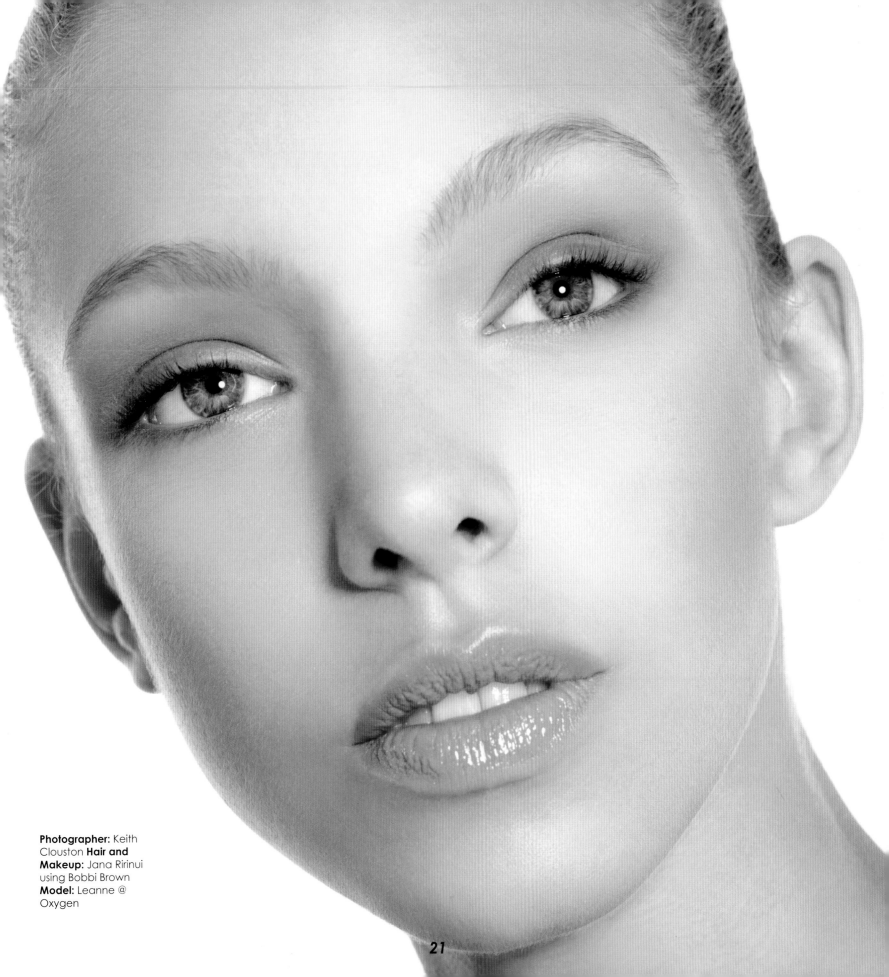

Photographer: Keith Clouston **Hair and Makeup:** Jana Ririnui using Bobbi Brown **Model:** Leanne @ Oxygen

Applying Foundation

1 Before applying foundation, make sure the skin is cleansed and moisturized. Wait a few minutes for the moisturizer to settle into the skin before application. If the face is damp and sticky, it can cause the foundation to clog up and look uneven. Try to use a non-sticky lotion that is not greasy or use a facial oil, such as Bio Oil.

2 Dab a small amount of foundation on the face in little dots on the forehead, down the nose and on the chin and cheeks.

3 Always apply in downward strokes to minimize pores. Sweep over ears and under jaw and do not cover up natural freckles or rosy cheeks.

4 Blend the foundation with a brush, sponge or your fingertips. Make sure it is blended completely to create a natural, flawless look. Always apply foundation quickly and lightly. Smooth, even strokes will prevent the colour looking clogged.

5 Check application in natural light to make sure the foundation is properly blended. If you need more coverage, apply concealer in specific areas rather than adding more foundation.

Concealing Dark Circles

Use a yellow-tinted concealer to hide dark purple circles and mauve or tan concealers to hide brownish circles; mauve or tan are also best for blending into dark or black skin. There are even green and light blue products to conceal red under-the-eye circles.

1 Apply several dots of concealer under the eyes, then tap and press in using your finger, never rub. Apply concealer on other uneven spots on the face – including the chin, and around the nose and mouth if need be – and tap in.

2 Pay close attention to the area where your eye meets the bridge of your nose. This area tends to have the darkest circles and consequently may need more concealer.

3 Apply foundation you normally wear to even out your complexion. Blend it as you usually would, without paying any special attention to under the eye. Once your foundation is in place, you should be able to clearly see any dark circles still evident. Then tap in a heavier coverage of concealer as in step 1.

4 Powder the concealed areas with a translucent powder, using just enough so that the concealer no longer looks sticky or shiny. Using a soft brush helps application.

• For more staying power and better coverage, let the concealer set for five to ten seconds after application and before blending.

• Mix a highlighter with the concealer to add brightness under the eye or use a brightening concealer. It will camouflage like a concealer, while adding flattering highlights to the face.

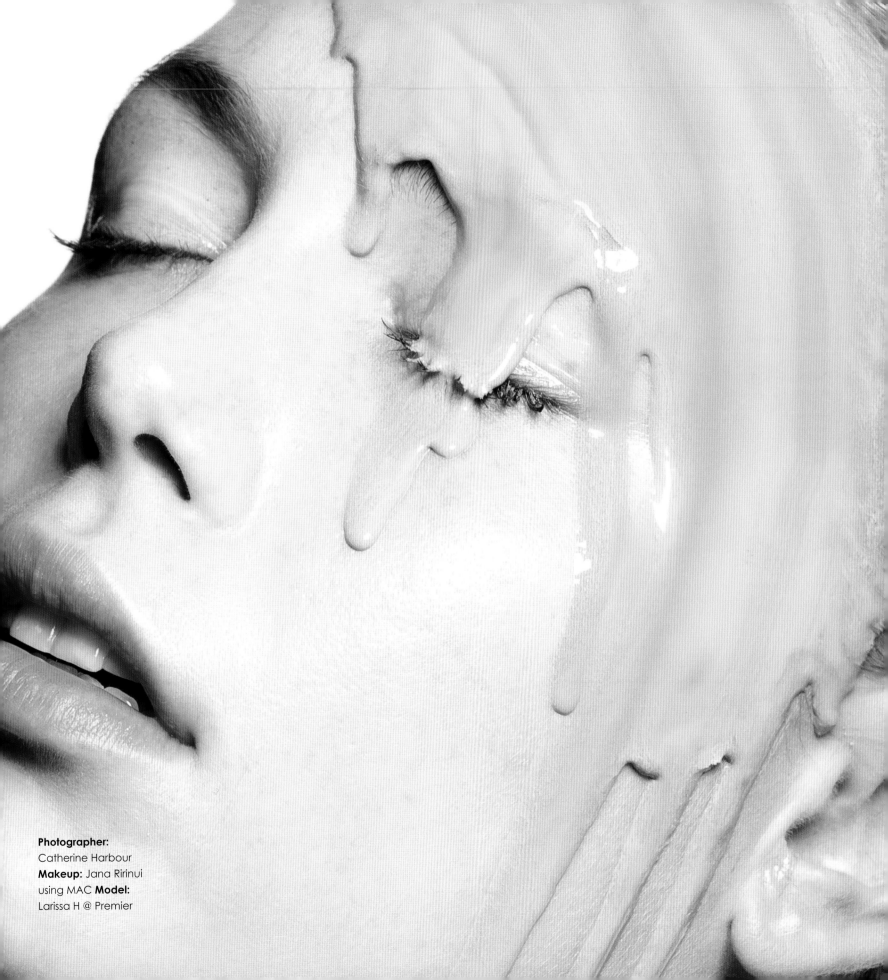

Photographer:
Catherine Harbour
Makeup: Jana Ririnui
using MAC **Model:**
Larissa H @ Premier

FOUNDATIONS & SKIN TONES

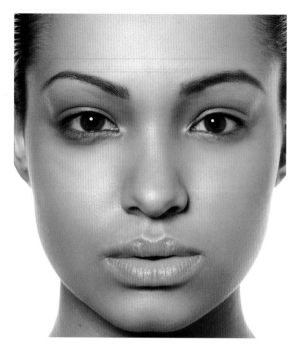

Photographer: Catherine Harbour **Makeup:** Ian Nguyen using Giorgio Armani **Model:** Naiyana

Photographer: Keith Clouston **Makeup:** Lan Nguyen using Giorgio Armani **Model:** Yu @ Oxygen

Matching makeup to skin tone is a tricky business. The perfect base foundation should even up the skin and highlight its natural radiance. Olive skin and dark skin naturally glows and rarely requires much concealer. It is important not to get stuck using the same makeup all year round as skin changes with the season and can be either dry or oily. It also gets slightly darker in the summer, then paler in the winter. Also in summer, the face and neck can be different colours where the sun catches the face rather than the neck. So it is a good idea to match the foundation to the neck or add a bronzer to even up the skin after you have finished your makeup application.

Ethnic women commonly have oily skin. Oil-control products work well, but skin tends to dry out if they are used on a regular basis. This is because these products typically contain alcohol. By matching the product to your skin type you can limit this problem.

Dark Skin Tones

Black skin has a tendency to become dull, grey and ashy-looking with the wrong foundation. It is also very rare for black or dual heritage skin to be uniform all over – darker foreheads, lighter cheekbones, and so on. Concealer should only be used if there are imperfections like scars, acne and large pores. It is extremely important to apply powder over foundation to set it and stop shine, rather than apply a heavy foundation. Other ways to limit shine are to use an oil-free primer before adding foundation and applying foundation with a brush or sponge instead of your fingers.

For dark skins, foundation should be somewhere between the natural skin colour and half a shade above or below. Use a tone-on-tone foundation or tinted moisturizer and add colour by using a blush or bronzer. It is best to choose a blush that highlights the skin tone, like peach, apricot, tan or even bronze, instead of the rosy pinks that are more suitable for pale skin. Layer the blush with more than one colour for a more dynamic look, using cream or powder blush. Shimmer on under-eye circles and wrinkles can be used lightly to brighten and contour the cheeks.

Latin, Indian and Asian Skin Tones

These skin tones are more olive-toned, so makeup with yellow undertones works best. Be forewarned that foundations sometimes turn a shade darker on oily skin because it mixes with the skin's natural oils; a lighter shade can be used to avoid foundation looking too dark. If cheeks have a natural, pink warmth, just dust a little powder (with pink undertones) on top of the foundation.

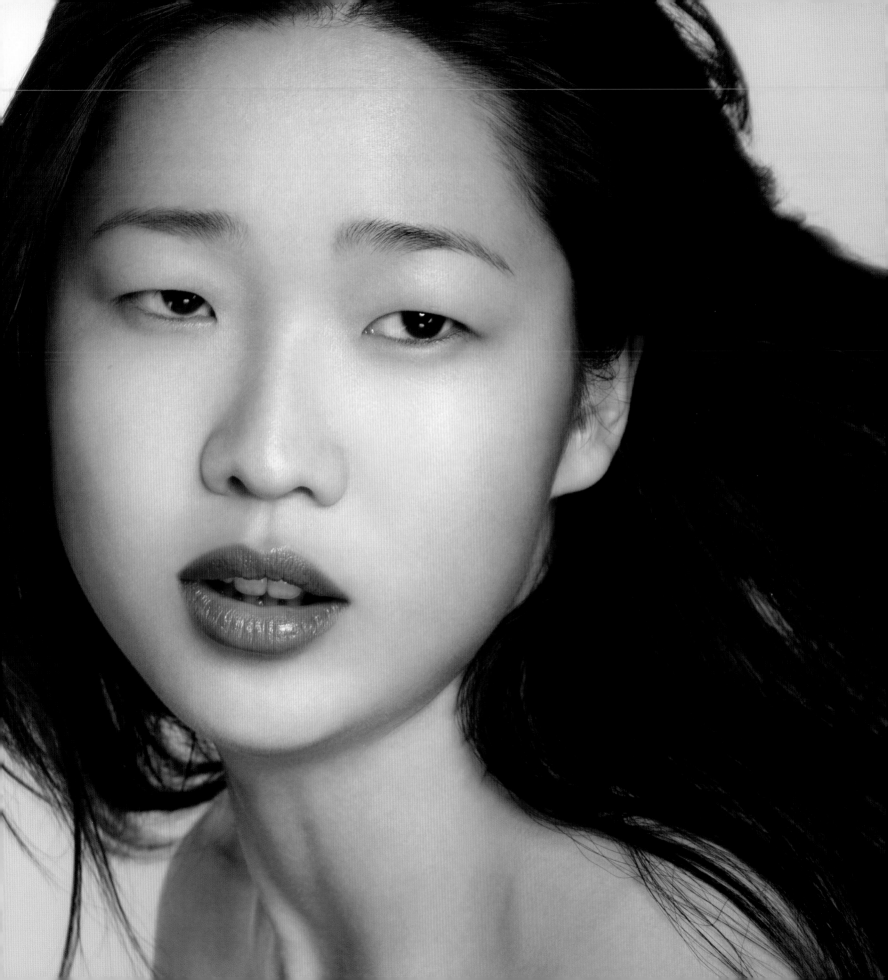

HIGHLIGHTING

Highlighting products are essential to help sculpt and contour the face. Whereas contour colours are used to create shadow and depth (see pages 32–3), highlighting products are used to reflect light, which adds an additional dimension of definition to the face. Highlighting is particularly popular in the fashion industry, in both editorial and catwalk shoots, where makeup is used to tell stories, create illusions and complement the fashion designer's vision.

Highlighting products come in a range of different textures, from shimmer powders and cream sticks to liquids and gels. There are different names for these products, including illuminizers, shimmers, iridescent and pearlized powders, but they all do the same thing.

An illuminizer (such as the Becca's Shimmering Skin Perfector) is great when mixed with a foundation to create a dewy, radiant glow and to even out skin tone. A slightly bronzed illuminzer mixed with foundation can add a subtle, bronzed, healthy glow.

Shimmer powder or liquids placed above the cheekbone reflect light and further enhance cheekbones. The Yves Saint Laurent Touche Éclat was originally designed for use as an illuminizer, but has proved popular as a concealer for under the eye. The highlighting effect reflects light and brightens dark circles.

Applying shimmer in a straight line down the centre of the nose creates the illusion of a straighter, smaller nose. Highlighters can also be applied to the centre of the lips to create the illusion of plumped, fuller lips.

On the catwalks, cream shimmers are often applied to the face first, then a powder shimmer is applied on top to create a strong, reflective effect. Highlighting is not just restricted to the face, but can also be used on the body to create the illusion of longer, more slender limbs. Highlighters can be brushed on to the collarbones and down the arms and the centre of the shins to give the illusion of length. Alternatively, oils can be used on the body to create a more reflective "wet" shine. MAC Strobe Cream is a popular choice for highlighting the body and can be mixed in with foundations.

Photographer: Zoe Barling **Makeup:** Sandra Cooke using Giorgio Armani **Hair:** Natasha Mygdal using Bumble & Bumble **Model:** Emma C @ IMG

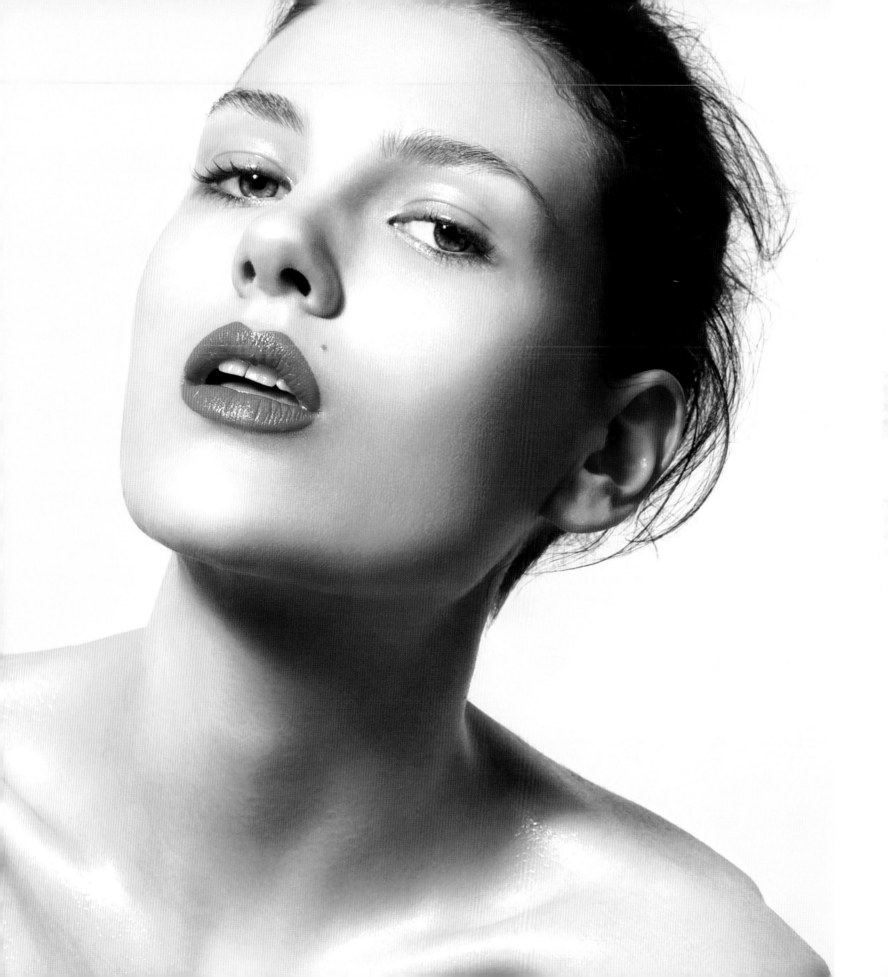

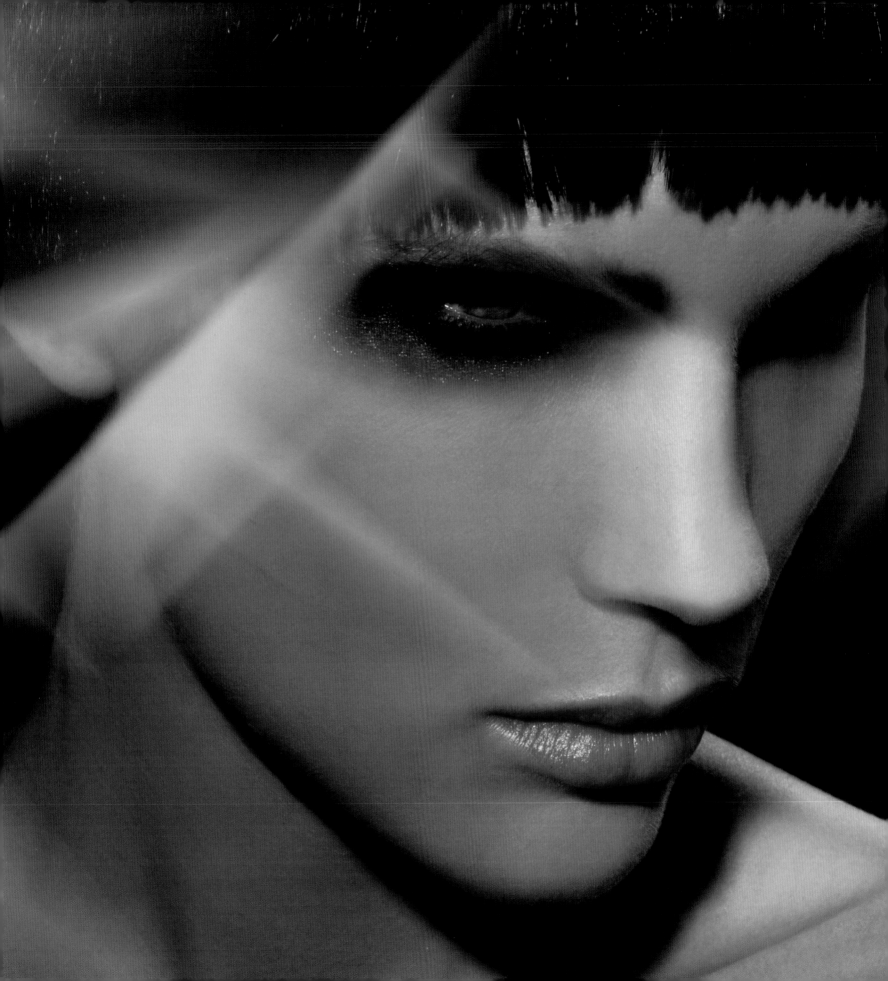

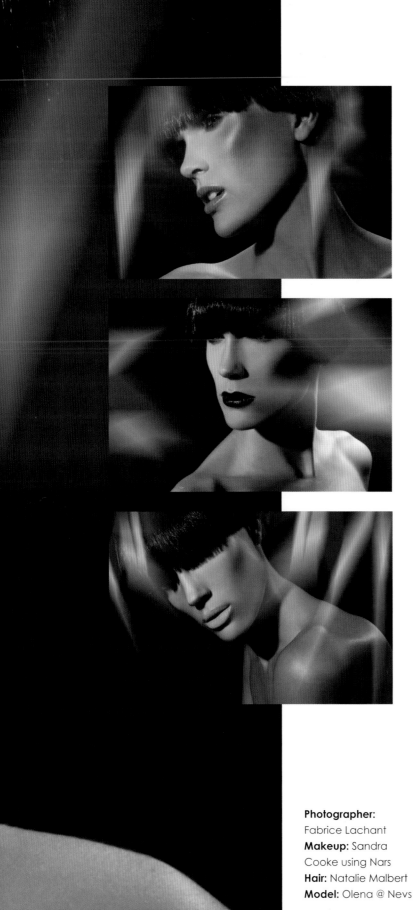

Blusher is the one product that can instantly make you look younger, healthier and prettier. A good blusher replaces the natural colours in your cheeks that drain away with age.

There are two types: cream and powder. Recently cosmetic brands have developed sculpting blushers that can be combined to create a strong and contoured cheekbone. Some powder blushes can be highly pigmented so you end up with excess product on the brush and it can look overdone, especially if placed too near to the nose.

Blushers can also be used for contouring, as can a wide range of products, such as eyeshadows, bronzers, and liquid and cream foundations, depending on the result you want to achieve. MAC cosmetics produce a range of sculpt and shading colours in the form of blushers that are specifically designed for contouring. The colours are all various shades of matte brown, cream and nude and are very much staples in a makeup artist kit.

Black and white photo shoots require clever use of contouring and highlighting, as the contrast of light and dark shadows affect the tone and shade of the makeup. Cool colours will seem lighter than they are and warm colours will appear grey and darker. Black pencil liner or eyeshadow will look dark grey, so a generous application is needed.

Photographer:
Fabrice Lachant
Makeup: Sandra
Cooke using Nars
Hair: Natalie Malbert
Model: Olena @ Nevs

Blushers

For healthy, natural colour, nothing beats blusher. However, it tends to be overused. Powder blush is typically best for oily and combination skin. Cream is great for dry skin and liquid and gel are best for oily skin. For even better results, combine cream and powder together – it helps blusher to stay on longer and looks more luminous. Cream blush is great for mature skin as it blends easily for a very natural look. Blush stains are ideal for well-moisturized skin but best avoided on dry skin as they tend to dry very fast. Blending cream blushers with a powder blush can also look very effective and beautiful on the skin.

Choosing a Colour

Start by choosing a colour, using nature as your guide. Find a colour that matches your cheeks when they are flushed after exercise or from being out in the cold. Fair skin looks great in rose, olive in peach and dark skin in apricot or even red. A dusky pink blusher will warm up any tired-looking skin. Another trick is to find one that matches your lip colour.

Applying Blusher

For best results, the skin should be prepped and foundation applied carefully. Apply the blush onto the high apple of the cheekbones and softly blend backward, following the cheekbone and ending at the hairline. Use a professional full brush for applying powder blush, tapping off any excess. For extra contouring and a more chiselled look, a bronzed or darker colour can be used underneath.

Blush should never go below the bottom of your nose or any closer in to the centre of your face than the iris of your eye. Apply a small amount of blush to your forehead – on the spot where the sun normally hits the face – if you look very pale. Applying blush near the eye can help give your eyes a sparkle, too.

- For over-applied powder blush, use translucent powder on top to calm down the colour. For over-applied cream blush, blot colour off with a tissue.

Applying Gels and Creams

For a natural, healthy flush, keep the colour light and blended. Dab a dot of gel or cream on the apple of the cheeks only, using the middle finger, then blend with ring and middle fingers. The clean finger will pick up any excess.

- A little foundation can be used to lighten over-applied gel or liquid blush, but as these formulas "stain" the cheeks, the only real way to correct the colour is to wash the face, moisturize and reapply.

Sun-Kissed Look

For a sun-kissed sheen dab bronzer powder on your forehead, chin and nose before applying a blush using a large brush and light strokes. Those with darker skin tones should try a caramel-coloured bronzer and avoid orange. After applying the blusher, use a sheer highlighting powder in a C-shape from the centre of your browbone to the centre of your cheeks. You can also dab a little shimmery blush on the highest point of the cheekbone, nearest the eye.

Working with Face Shapes

Accentuate the cheekbones by using a slightly darker shade in that area, while blending it down the cheek for a more natural look. If you have a full face, focus your blush near your hairline. If you have high cheekbones, apply the blush to in the centre of your face and do not apply to the underside of your cheeks.

Round faces: Give an illusion of slenderness by applying blush in a sideways V on the cheekbones. Blend it well and add a little to the chin as well.

Square faces: Soften the square angles of the face with a dab of blush on the forehead and chin. Apply blush from the centre of the eyes toward the cheekbones and blend.

Rectangular faces: Applying blush below the outer corners of the eyes will reduce the elongated square shape.

Oval faces: Apply blush to the prominent part of the cheekbone and blend it carefully toward the temples.

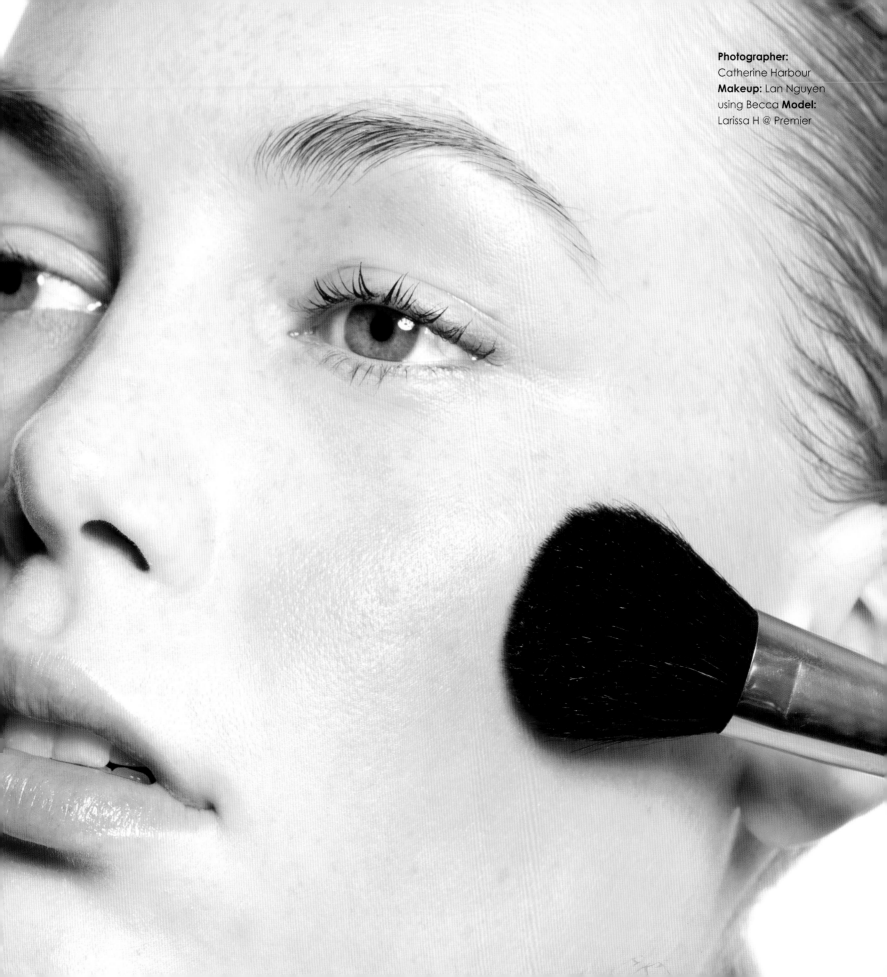

Photographer:
Catherine Harbour
Makeup: Lan Nguyen
using Becca **Model:**
Larissa H @ Premier

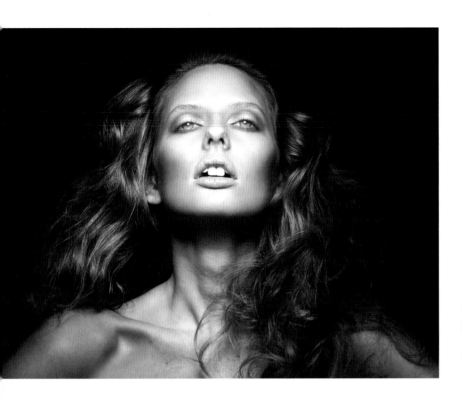

Photographer:
Roberto Aguilar
Makeup: Sandra Cook
using MAC **Hair:** Heath
Grout using Tigi **Model:**
Darya @ FM Models

Contouring

Contouring creates illusions on the face. It is the art of using shadow and highlight to sculpt, emphasize and accentuate features. A prime example of this is with cheekbones: highlighting above the bone and shadowing just below dramatically draws out the cheekbone.

To truly understand contouring, you need to understand the structure of the face. Symmetry is actually what makes a face "beautiful" and more photogenic, and so contouring can be used as a tool to create the illusion of balance and symmetry in the face. Even the most subtle form of contouring has the power to transform, creating a natural look without the need to add colour and "makeup". Contouring can also be done on a far more obvious level, particularly in high fashion where it is a deliberate feature of the makeup. Contouring can do the following:

* Give more defined cheekbones.
* Define the jawline/chin and minimize a "double" chin.
* Minimize a large forehead.
* Create fuller lips.
* Straighten and/or narrow a wider/larger nose.
* Lift sagging eyes.

• The key point to remember is that the dark colours draw back and make things appear smaller and lighter colours make features appear larger and closer.

• Always use a matte shade when creating shadows. For achieving a natural contour look, this should be between two and three shades darker than the skin tone.

• You can use a matte or shimmer product to highlight, although for more mature skins it is recommended that a matte shade is used, as shimmer products will accentuate fine lines and wrinkles.

• The level of blending you do will determine how natural the contouring looks. Always check all angles of your face in a natural light before completion, to ensure there are no obvious streaks.

• Highlighting is the opposite of contouring. With darker shades, you create a shadow, such as under the cheekbone, to help create the "shape", whereas the highlight colour, applied where the light would hit the bone – above the cheekbone, not on the cheekbone, helps create the "depth" of the shape.

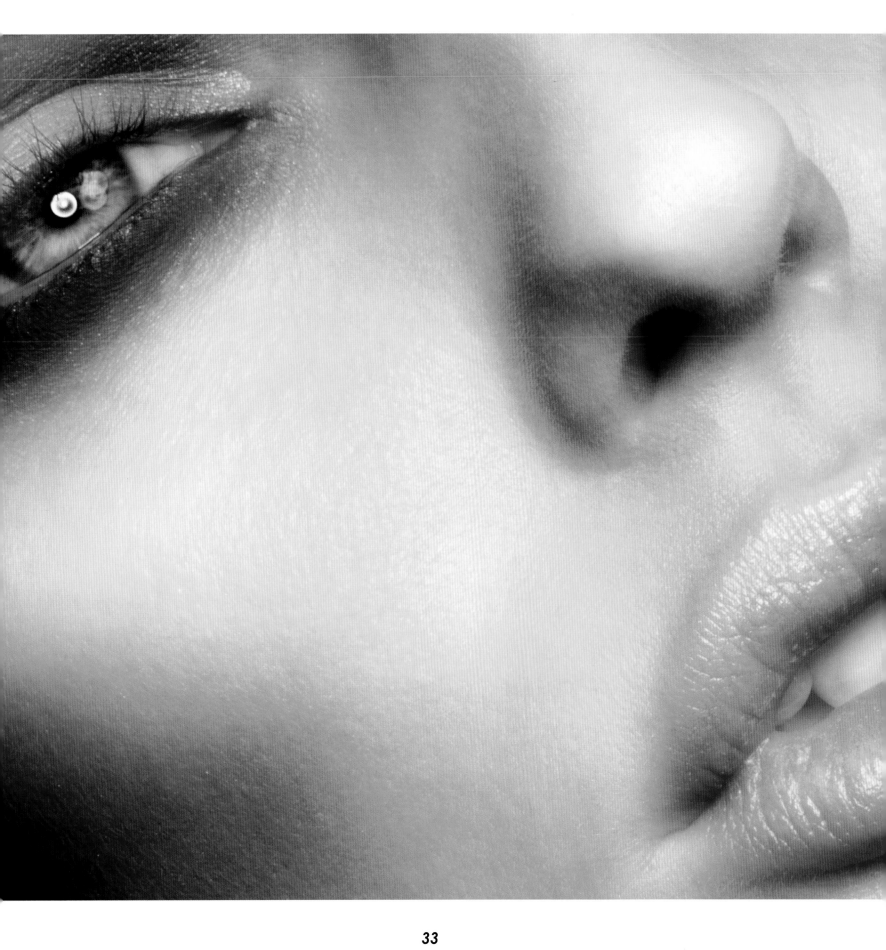

POWDERS

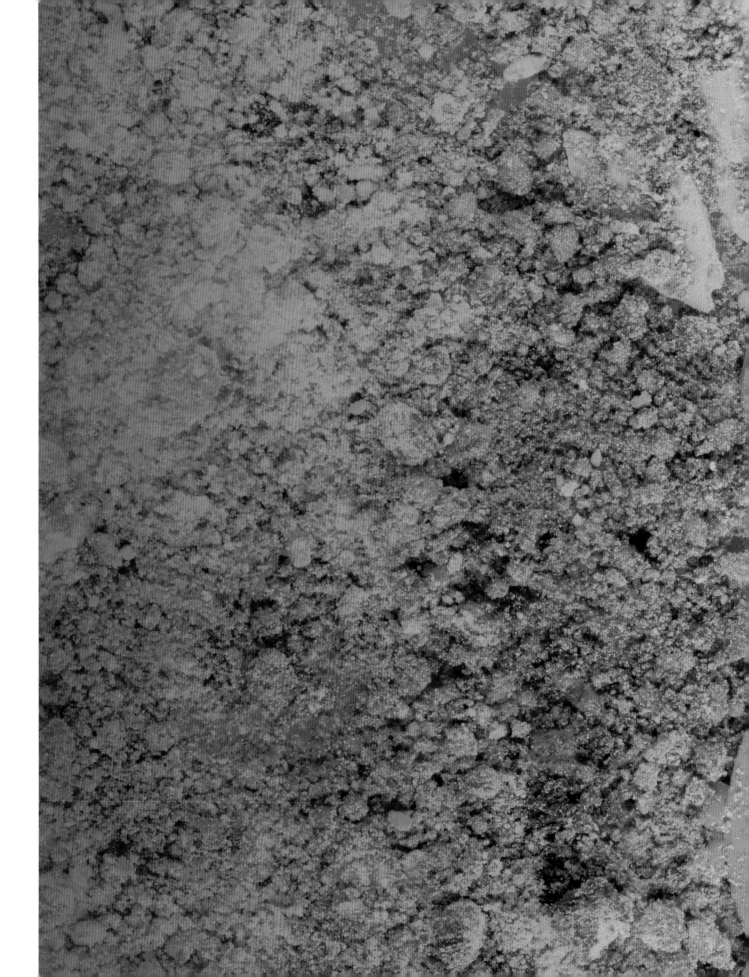

Photographer:
Camille Sanson

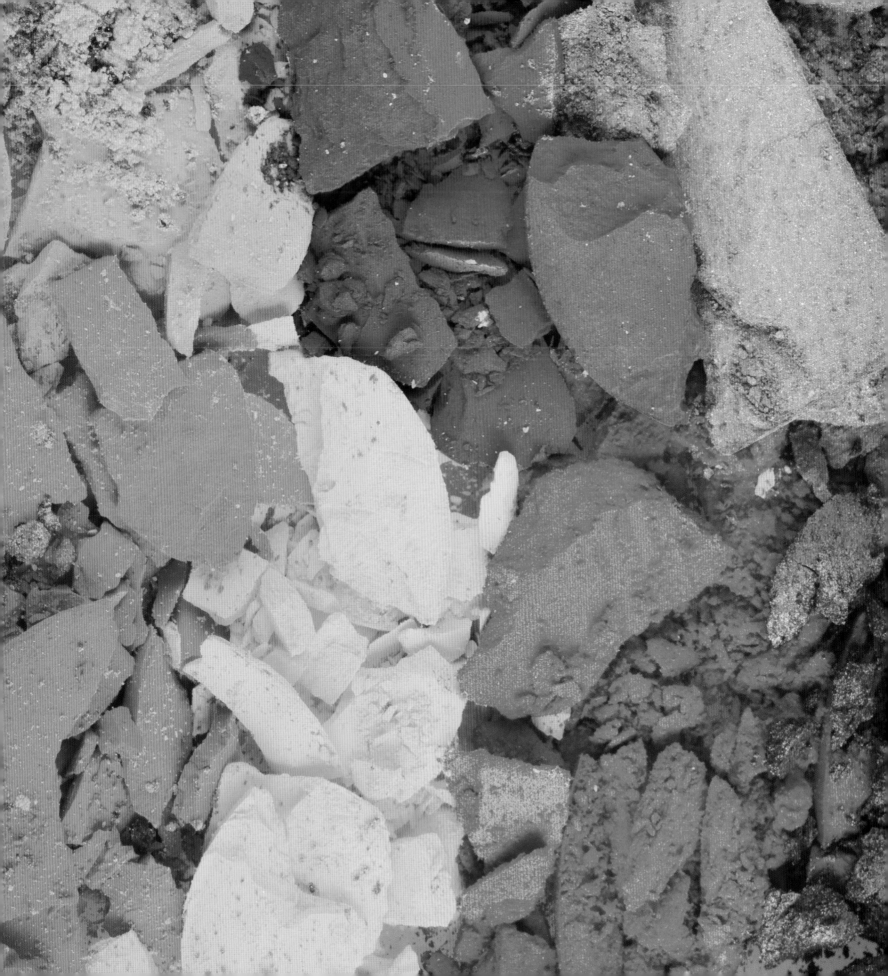

Sheer and Translucent Powders

There are many different types of powder, ranging from pressed to loose powders and sheer to full coverage. The suitability of each depends on whether you are using it for everyday wear, bridal, fashion/editorial or television and film. Sheer powders or blot powders are great for setting foundation and reducing shine on the skin. The nice thing about them is that they tend not build up or get "cakey" after a few applications. This makes them great for all-day shoots or everyday wear. You may also use loose translucent powder, which gives a sheer finish. A colourless powder can be used on a wide range of skin tones from dark to light. A good one is the matte Shu Uemura loose powder, as the particles are very fine and absorb a maximum amount of oil on the skin.

- You can use a dark-coloured sheer powder as a bronzer on lighter tones of skin.

Coverage Powders

You can also purchase powders with a bit more coverage to them. These are useful to take out any redness in the skin or level out skin tone. MAC Mineralize Skin Finish powders are great for this, as they melt right into the skin and even out any discoloration. If you have a slightly incorrectly coloured foundation, these powders can deepen the skin tone or lighten it up a shade, depending on what colour is used.

There are full-coverage powders on the market as well. These can be used like a foundation. Some people prefer to use these (as opposed to liquid foundation) because they are faster to apply and easier to carry around for touching up. They are good for the everyday person, but would be far too heavy to use constantly on a bride or during a photo shoot.

You can get away with coverage powders as a "quick fix" backstage if a model needs a bit more coverage before she heads out on the catwalk. A popular full coverage powder is Studio Fix by MAC.

Loose and Pressed Powders

For the everyday person, the choice between loose and pressed powder is usually down to personal preference. Things to consider are whether or not you will need to be carrying it around for touch-ups (in which case a loose powder can be more bulky and messy) and what kind of coverage you would like to get out of a powder, as most loose powders tend to be more sheer in style.

Backstage at a fashion show, pressed powders are usually preferred. This is because they are far less messy to run around with and it is less likely the powder will spill or blow onto the clothes. During a fashion or editorial shoot, the choice of powders can be left to the artist's preference. Here, they will have more space and hopefully a station, so there will be less worries about being bumped into and spilling powder on the clothes.

- Wait to powder the face of your model on the shoot until the photographer has taken the first shot. This is because you may not need to powder the face at all, depending on what type of look you are going for, or you may only need minimal powder in certain areas.

- At a wedding, a pressed powder may be more beneficial as you can carry it around easily all day and evening for touch-ups. If you are not staying around for the full day, you can give the powder to the bride so she can use it herself without worrying about making a mess.

Photographer:
Catherine Harbour
Makeup: Lan Nguyen
using Shu Uemura
Model: Larissa H @
Premier

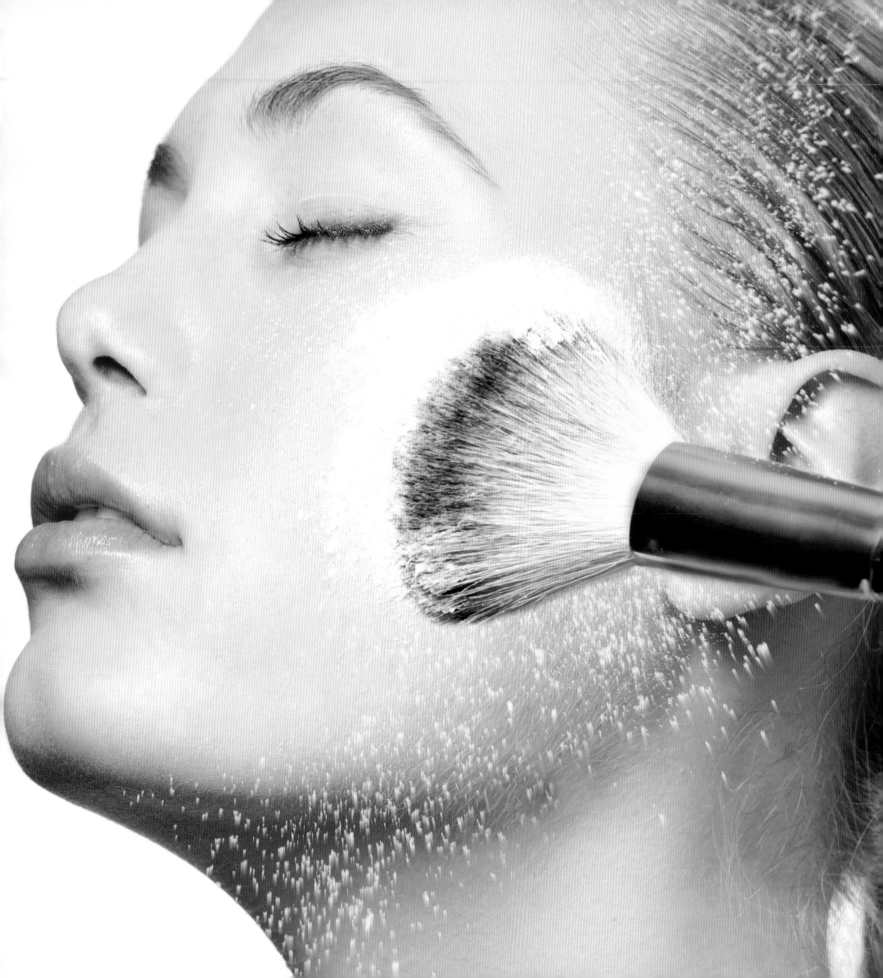

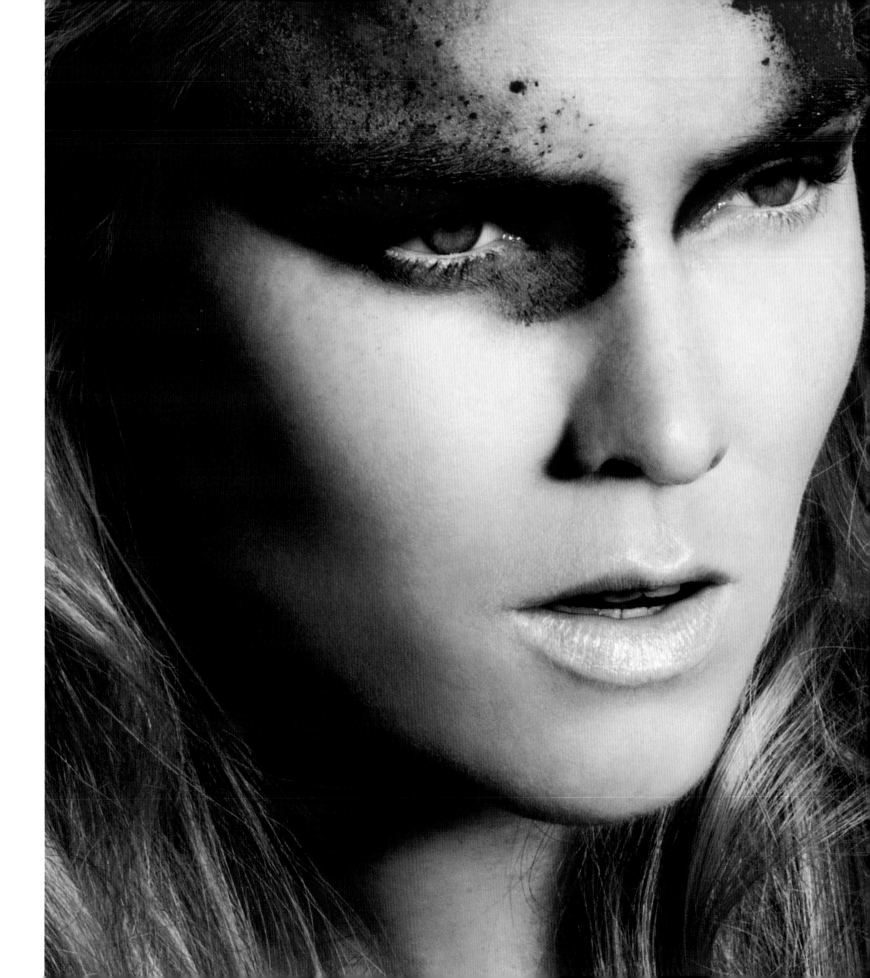

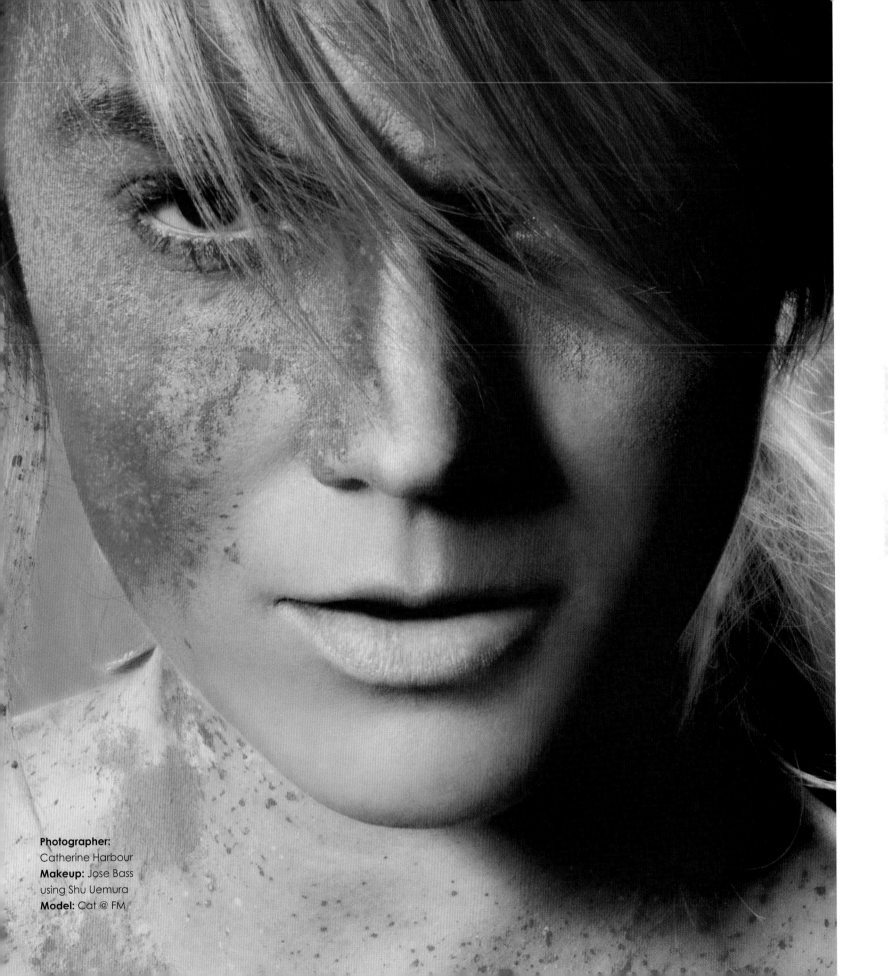

Photographer:
Catherine Harbour
Makeup: Jose Bass
using Shu Uemura
Model: Cat @ FM

Being tanned or bronzed gives people a healthy glow that is generally associated with a relaxing holiday in the sun. It also gives the appearance of being slimmer and helps hide skin imperfections. However, people are now aware, more than ever, that real tans can prematurely age skin and cause skin cancer – hence the beauty industry's fascination with fake tanning products.

There are so many products available that give a good tan effect that there is no excuse for anybody to go out and soak up the sun and burn their skin. The colour choices are vast and suit everyone from the whitest of white to olive skin tones. They do require a little effort, but in the long term they will save your skin and allow you to walk round with a year-long healthy glow.

Temporary Bronzing

Considering spring/summer fashion collections are shot during the winter, makeup artists need to use a great deal of fake tans and bronzers. On a photo shoot, artists have a number of options to tan the skin. An airbrush machine can be used to apply temporary tans to models. Alcohol-based airbrush paints do not rub off on clothes or in water. Instead, they are quick to dry, and can easily be applied with a compressor and a specialized body air gun. This process, however, can be messy and requires specialist equipment, product and remover.

To create that sun-kissed glow without an air gun, the makeup artist has a variety of different products to consider. At fashion week it is common to see makeup artists using body foundation, often mixed with moisturizer, to cover blemishes and darken the legs, arms, back and any other skin showing on the models. There are also numerous bronzing products available, such as bronzed oils, gels, lotions and creams, that all provide an instant tan, but which can easily be washed off at the end of a shoot. These kinds of product are not ideal to use with certain clothes as they can stain. Powdered bronzers are also great, but are generally better used on smaller areas, such as the face and chest, rather than the whole body. Shimmer bronzers can also be used to accentuate and highlight points, such as the front of the shins, thighs, shoulders and collar bone.

For those wishing to be bronzed for a special one-off event, there are numerous body and face bronzers that will wash off with water at the end of the night. The only downside with this option is that if it is extremely hot or raining, your beautiful healthy glow may run off or, even worse, cause streaks! Bronzers can also tend to get on clothes, although as most are water-based, they are easily washed off. For makeup artists, bronzers are ideal for changing the skin tone on photo shoots, as it is quick, easy and can be applied exactly where it is needed.

Again, the bronzers come in a variety of different mediums, such as creams, lotions, sprays and powders. Facial bronzers can be very simply applied all over the face or, to give a realistic, sun-kissed glow, applied only on the places where the sun would fall, as it would if you were tanning naturally, along the cheek bones, temples, forehead and lightly along the length of the nose and the chin. This soft wash of colour will lift the face, giving an extra-healthy glow.

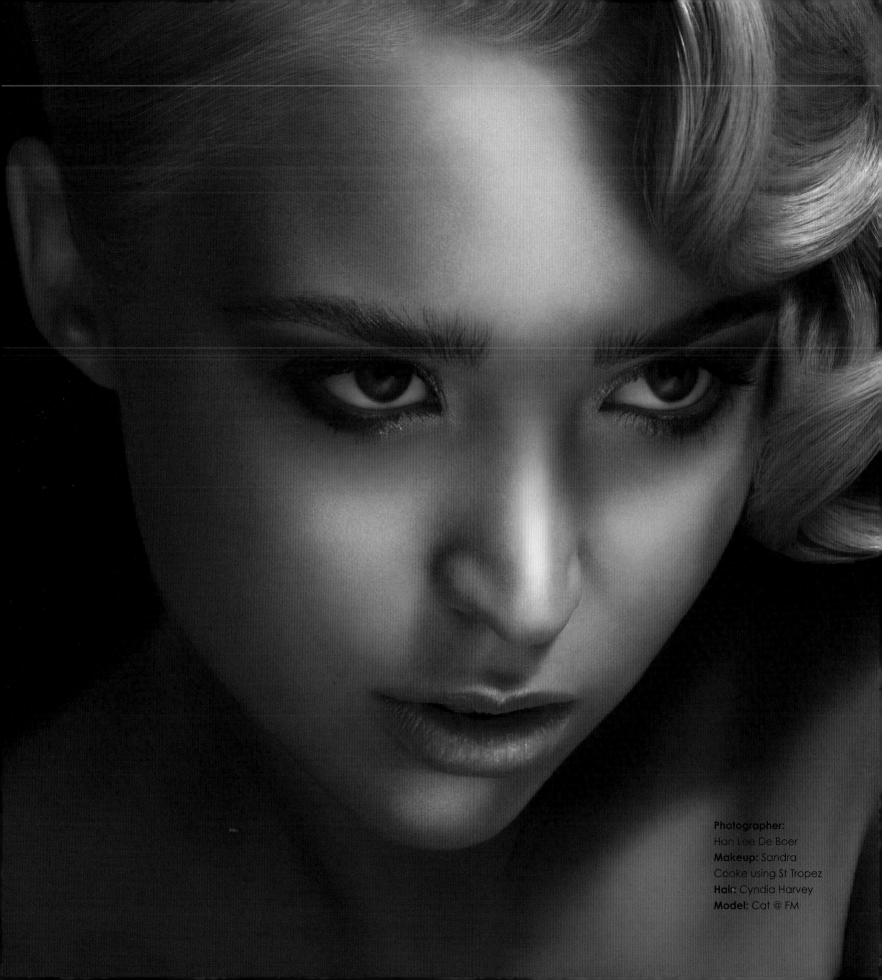

Photographer:
Han Lee De Boer
Makeup: Sandra
Cooke using St Tropez
Hair: Cyndia Harvey
Model: Cat @ FM

Lasting Fake Tans

For a lasting tan, the quickest and most efficient way to get that all-over bronzed glow is to get a spray tan, applied by a trained therapist using a spray gun. You can choose from a light golden glow to very dark tan and the colour is dependent on the number of coats you wish to have applied. Most tans will develop over a couple of hours. Prior to the tanning, it is recommend that a full-body exfoliation is done so that all rough skin is removed – this helps the colour go on evenly. Spray tans usually last about a week and can be maintained with proper body exfoliation and moisturizing, as well as weekly top-ups.

There are other at-home fake tan options, such as aerosol sprays, creams, gels and lotions. These can be messy and take time to dry, but they do provide a good alternative to the spray tan. The newest trend is the gradual tan – body moisturizers with a hint of fake tan that gradually build up to create and maintain a healthy glow.

Getting the Perfect Tan

Fake tans usually take between 2 to 4 hours to develop. Make sure you read the instructions for the particular product you are using, and always wait the recommended time before applying a second coat if you want to go darker.

1 To ensure an even, lasting tan, ensure any hair removal is done a day prior to application.

2 Before starting, exfoliate to ensure the skin is silky smooth.

3 Make sure drier areas, such as elbows, knees and ankles, are well moisturized to help avoid unsightly product buildup on these areas.

4 Apply the tan with a tanning mitt so as not to stain your hands and to create a more even coverage. You may need to get a friend to apply the product in hard-to-reach places.

5 Before the product dries, use a soft cloth to gently wipe the knees, ankles, elbows, and in between the fingers and toes to remove extra product, which tends to cling to these areas.

6 Wear old, loose clothing while you are waiting for the product to dry.

• To maintain your tan, top up the application about once a week. Participating in intense sports or water activities will reduce the life of your tan, and you may need to apply more coats more regularly.

• Try not to shower for 24 hours after application of the tan.

• Regular light exfoliation and moisturizing will help prolong and even the tan.

Photographer:
Roberto Aguilar
Makeup: Sandra
Cooke using St Tropez
Hair: Heath Grout
using Tigi **Model:** Darya
@ FM Models

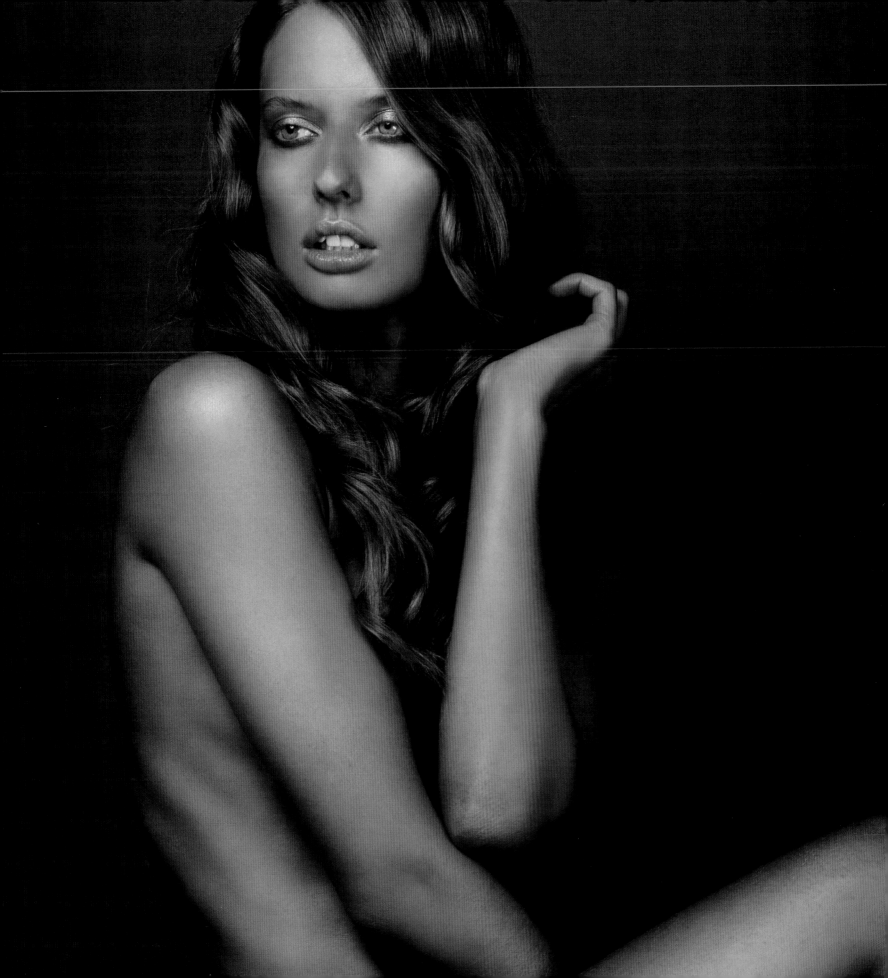

THE *EYES*

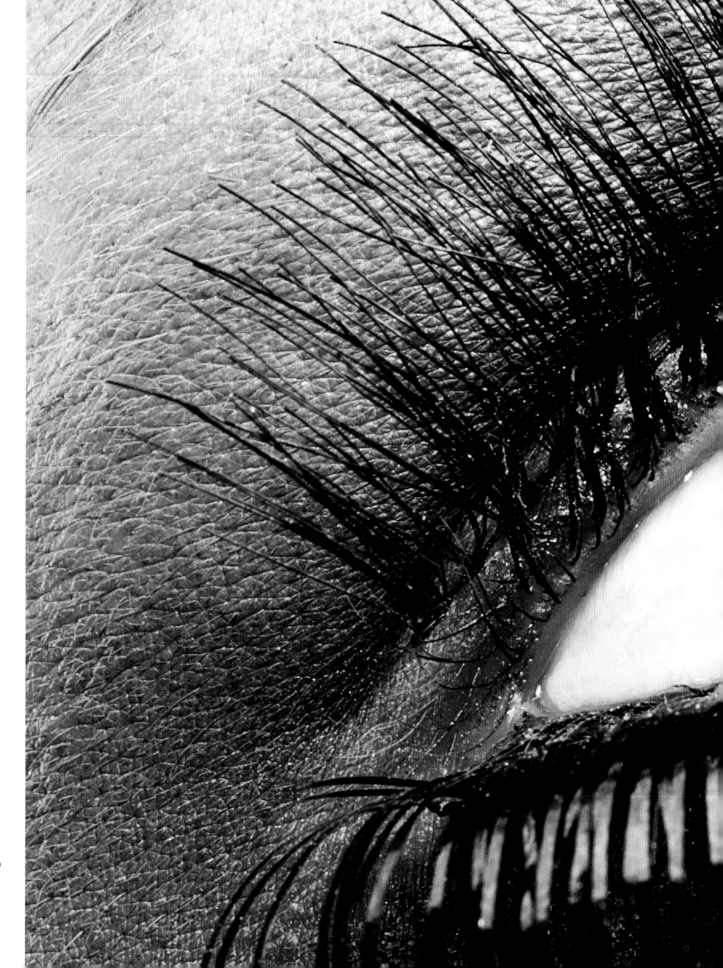

Photographer: Roberto Aguliar **Makeup:** Jose Bass using Shu Uemura

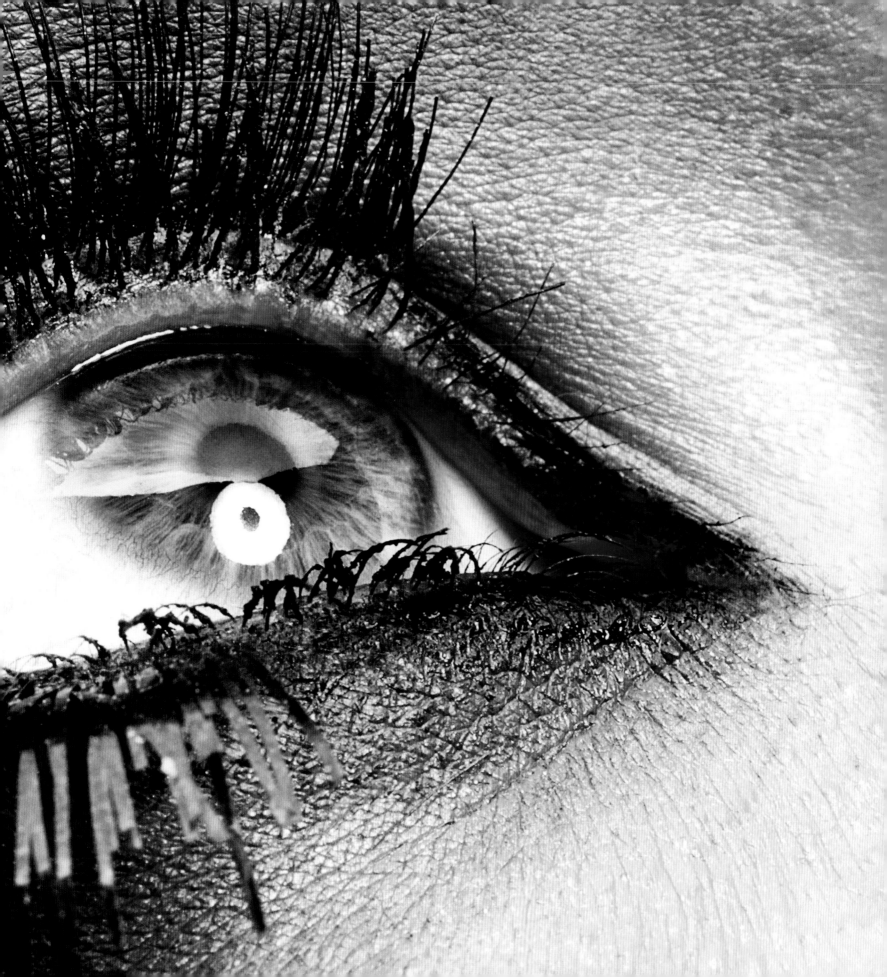

EYEBROWS

Eyebrows frame the face. Therefore, it is good to have them clean, visible and shaped to match the face. For a natural, symmetrical look, the length of the eyebrows must be slightly longer than the eye. This means that the brow needs to start just above the tear duct and end approximately 5mm (3/16 in) after the outer corner of the eye. This will create a young and fresh look.

Eyebrow Shaping

When it comes to the arch of the eyebrow be very careful to find the correct position of the arch. To do this, look straight into a mirror, place the handle of a thin makeup brush on the outside of your nostril and point it so that it is in line with the outside of your iris. Where the brush crosses the brow is where the highest point of the arch should be.

To define the brow, remove all the hairs on top of the eyebrow. If you are worried, imagine a straight line from the start of your eyebrow up to the highest point of the arch. All the hairs above this line are unnecessary so pluck them away. This will leave you with a sharp and defined brow shape.

Repeat the same process underneath the brow. Imagine a straight line from beneath to the highest point of the arch, everything under this line can be taken away. Be very careful as you pluck, just three hairs plucked away or left can make a huge difference.

Another way of shaping the eyebrows is to trim them. Where there is excess hair, or any hairs that are particularly unruly, brush them upward and trim off any length that goes over the imaginary lines mentioned previously. If your brows still need more definition, then you can apply a little brow shadow to outline the new defined shape. Use an ashy brown on lighter brows, and for really dark brows try a plum tone.

- If you want a cat-like look, make your brows longer and straighter – this is a great look for older women who want to look a little younger.

- If you want to disguise your own brow and draw on a completely new one, then a great tip is to wet some soap, apply it like a paste over the eyebrow and then carefully add a good concealer on top. You can then draw on any style of eyebrow that you want.

- The best way to get really good at styling eyebrows is to practice on paper – try drawing different styles and shapes.

- Avoid having the arch in the middle of the brow. It will make the eyes look narrow. By having the arch a little further along, the eyes will look open and full.

- Do not pluck the start of the brow too much, if the brows look too far apart from each other it will make the eyes look as if they are on the side of the head – like a fish!

- The best tweezers have pointy ends and only take one hair out at a time. Tweezers with a slanted edge will take lots of hairs out in one go, which can lead to over-plucking, resulting in the wrong shape brow.

Photographer: Allan Chiu **Makeup:** Jose Bass using Shu Uemura **Model:** Anna @ FM

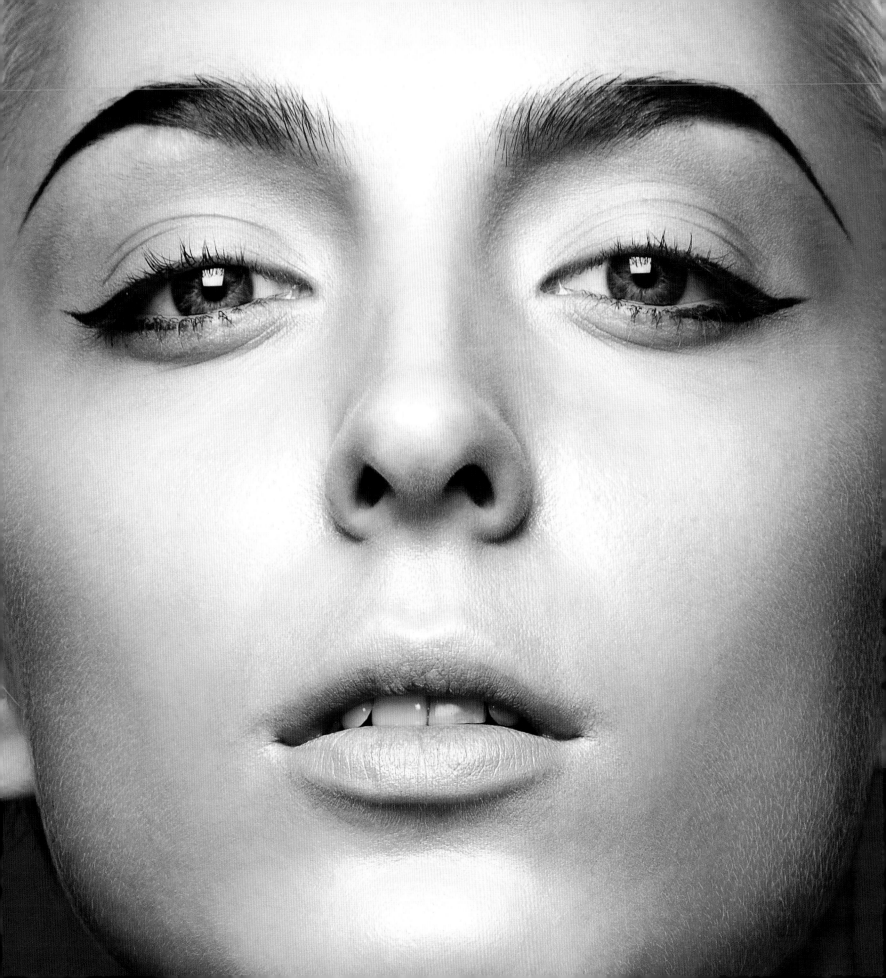

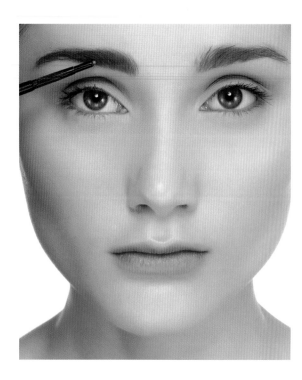

Enhancing Brows

To give shape and definition to the eyebrows it is as necessary to clear strays from above as it is from below the natural eyebrow. The widest part of the eyebrow should be the starting point in the centre, and it should get progressively thinner until the thinnest point at the end.

1 The eyebrow should be slightly longer than the outer corner of the eye. The starting point of the eyebrow should be aligned with your tear duct. Hold a thin makeup brush vertically alongside the nose to see a straight line from the tear duct to the start of the eyebrow.

2 The arch should normally be where the browbone stands out – the part of the eyebrow starting at the start and meeting the highest point should be longer than the part that stretches from the arch outward to the end. To find the ideal arch, angle a thin makeup brush from the side of your nose across the outer part of your iris. This will give you an idea where the arch should be.

3 To make shaping easier, draw in the eyebrows before plucking them. It is a good idea to first draw different brow shapes on a piece of paper. You can make the arch angle pointy, or more curvaceous and natural. Repeat this as much as you need to because it will help you visualize the eyebrow before drawing it onto the face. It will also ensure that you do not get distracted by the natural (or unnatural) shape of the eyebrows.

4 Once you have defined the line, draw in your eyebrows with an eyebrow pencil or eyebrow powder. A powder can be easily erased if you make a mistake.

5 Now pluck every hair above and below your drawn line.

6 If the hair is too long at the start of the brow, brush the hair directly upward and trim it to the top drawn line. Leave a tiny extra so you do not over-trim. Sometimes the hair at the end of the eyebrows is long and stubborn, in which case brush it down and trim it according to the line you have drawn.

7 To make the brows more defined and full, fill them in with powder and brush them softly to make them look natural. The result should be well-defined brows which draws more attention to a clean eye.

Photographer: Keith Clouston **Makeup:** Jade Hunka using Shu Uemura **Model:** Elena @ Oxygen

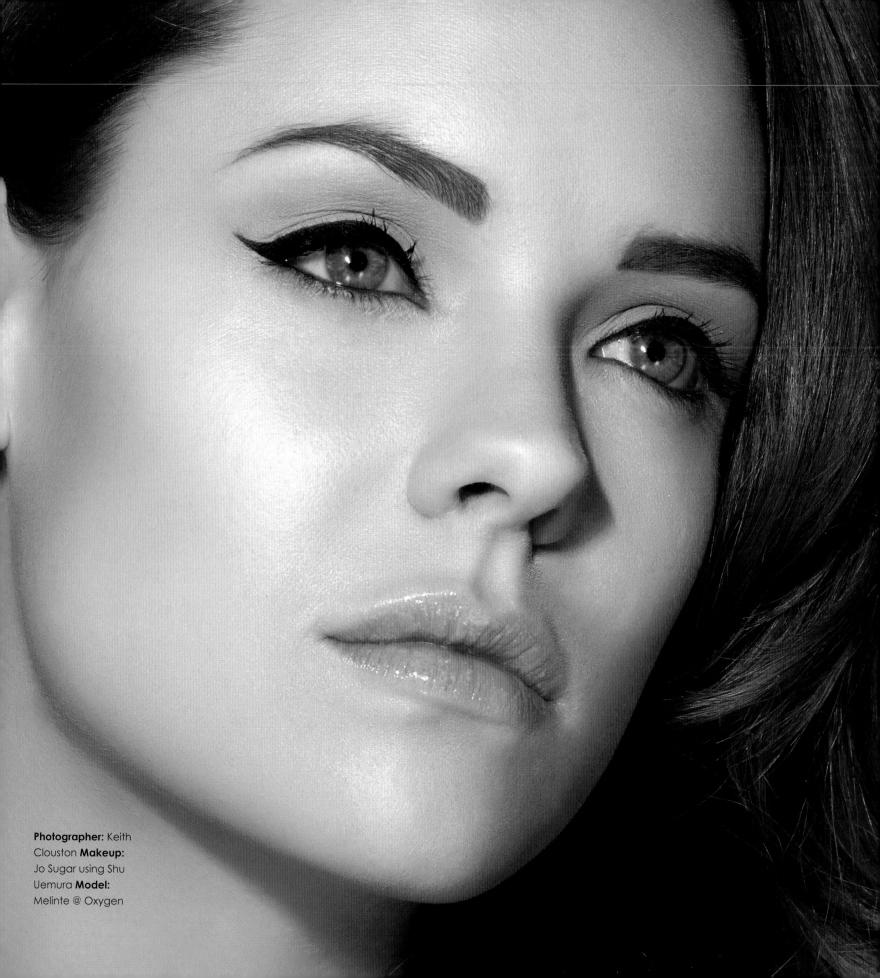

Photographer: Keith
Clouston Makeup:
Jo Sugar using Shu
Uemura Model:
Melinte @ Oxygen

EYESHADOW TEXTURES

How the colour of the eyeshadow appears on the eyelid depends on the cosmetic brand used, its texture and its application. Using an eye primer or eyeshadow base, such as Benefit's Lemon Aid, can boost colour, eliminate creasing and allow the makeup to last longer.

Matte

Matte eyeshadow is a flat colour without shine. It is a great choice as a contour or crease colour on a photo shoot, as it gives a better appearance of depth than shimmery shades. A contour eyeshadow brush is a useful tool to get this desired effect.

Cream

Cream shadows have a moist or wet texture. Some creams that stay moist and appear wet are prone to creasing, while others go on wet, but set dry. Bobbi Brown's Longwear cream shadow has a great crease-proof formula. Cream shadows also work well as a base on the eyelid to intensify the colour of a powder shadow.

Frost

Frost eyeshadow has a crystal-like shine to it. When applying it, use a stiff brush, which will give a stronger application of the frosted pigment.

Glitter

Containing small particles of sparkle to reflect light, glitters are great for music videos, pop promos and night shoots, as they add a real "wow" factor. Loose glitter can be applied on the eye area like an eyeshadow, but it needs a sticky surface to grip onto, such as a cream shadow or eyelash glue.

Loose Pigment

A loose-pigmented eyeshadow is made up of tiny particles of colour and usually comes in a small pot with a lid, rather than a flat casing. You can get varying degrees of effects with loose pigment shadow. If applied to the eye area with a fluffy brush, it can create a sheer wash of colour. If loose pigment is applied to the eyelid with a denser tool, such as a basic eyeshadow pad, then you get a more opaque and stronger tone. Loose pigment can also be mixed into a liquid, such as MAC's Mixing Medium to create a liquid makeup that can be painted onto the skin. Barry M's range of loose pigments come in a terrific colour palette.

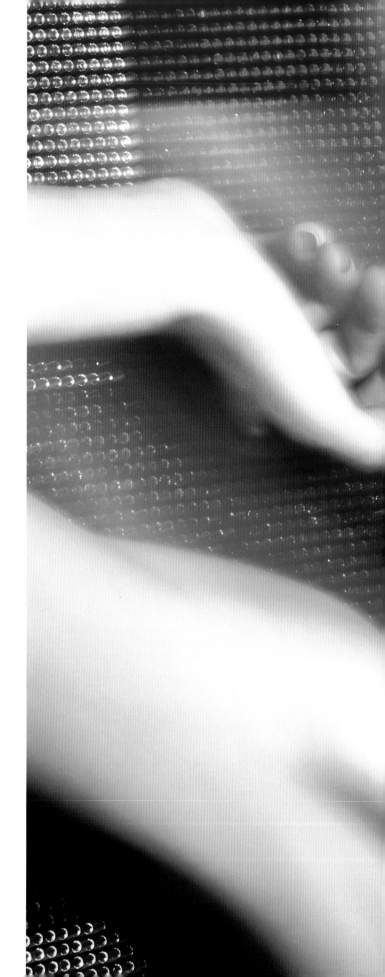

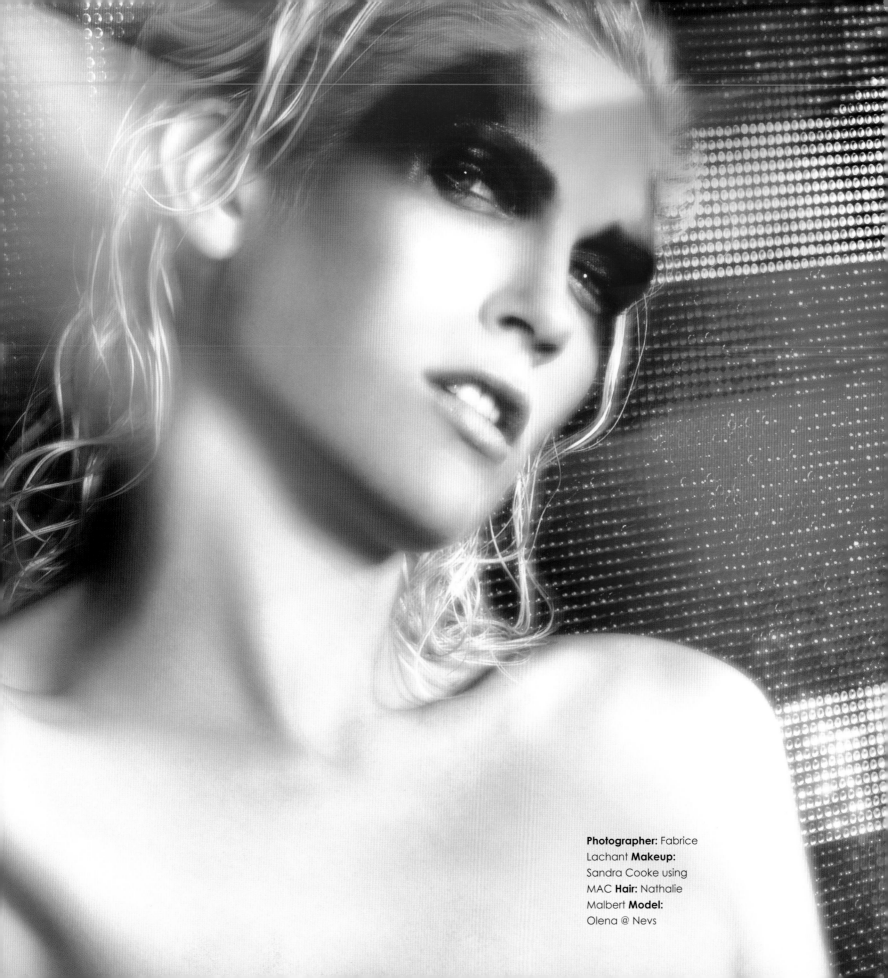

Photographer: Fabrice
Lachant **Makeup:**
Sandra Cooke using
MAC **Hair:** Nathalie
Malbert **Model:**
Olena @ Nevs

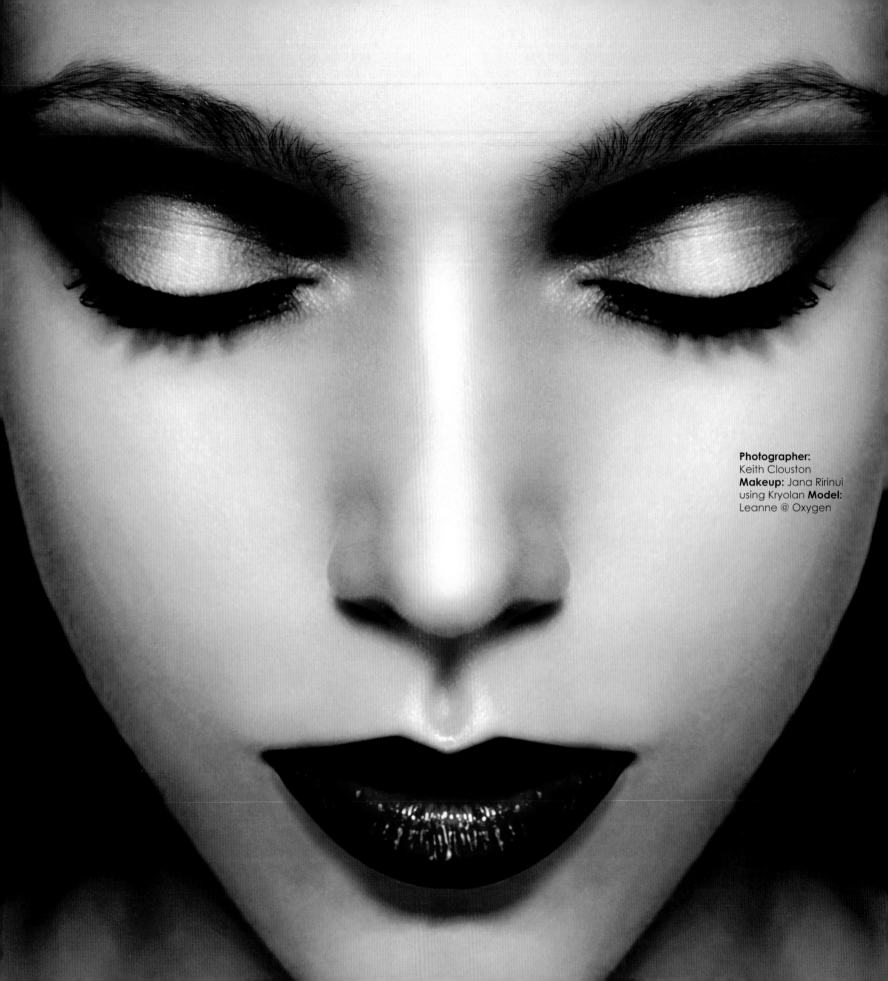

Photographer:
Keith Clouston
Makeup: Jana Ririnui
using Kryolan **Model:**
Leanne @ Oxygen

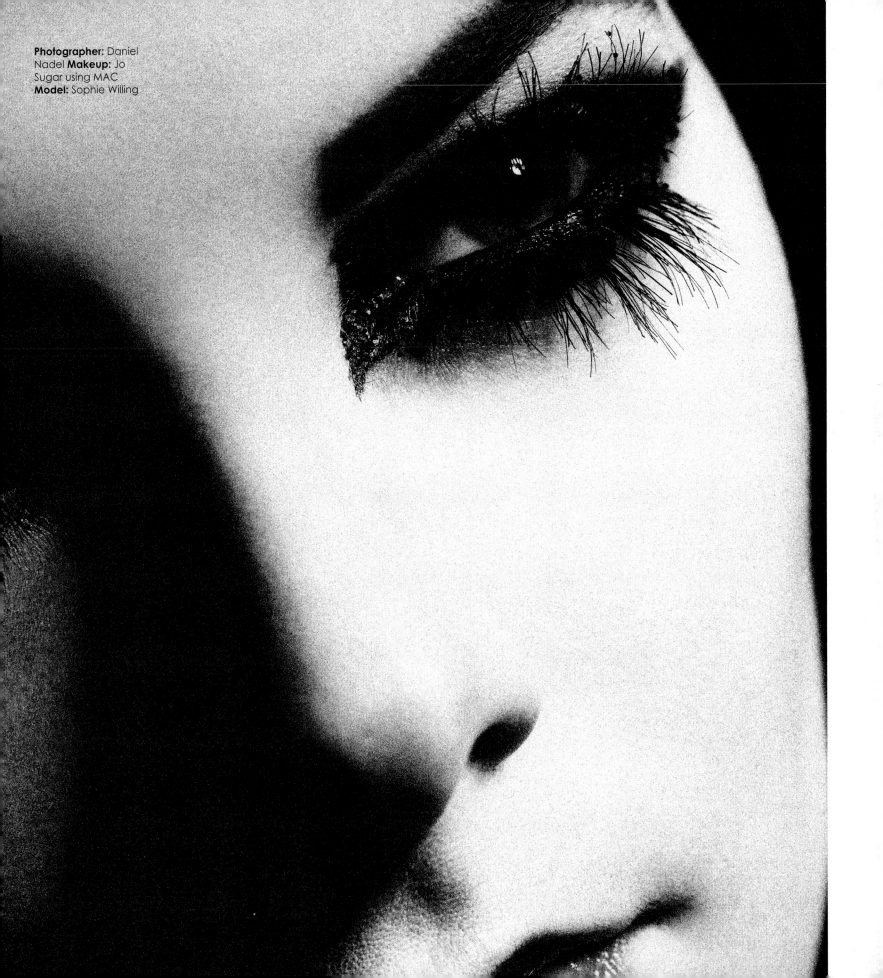

Photographer: Daniel Nadel **Makeup:** Jo Sugar using MAC **Model:** Sophie Willing

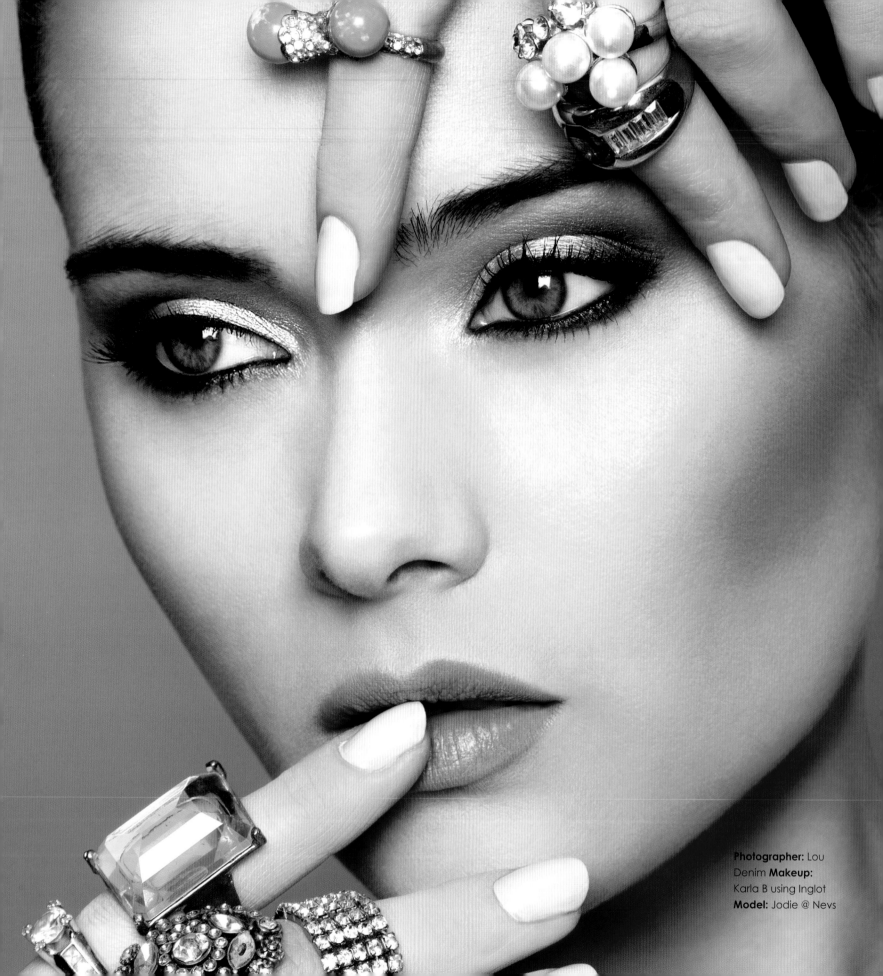

Photographer: Lou Denim **Makeup:** Karla B using Inglot **Model:** Jodie @ Nevs

There are many ways to create a smoky eye, but the most popular is by using black powder eyeshadow all the way around the eye and then blending upward and out above the crease. You can also use cream shadows, greasepaint or gel eyeliner. Once you have mastered the art of blending this bold look, you can start using strong colours or pigments and playing around with different shapes such as the "cat eye" (great for nights out), a "panda eye" (which is very trendy and grungy, see also page 85) and smokier eyes using cream shadow and a kohl pencil.

To create a good smoky eye, you must invest in quality brushes, but you will only need two. The first is an application brush to sweep on the eyeshadow, such as a Kolinsky sable-hair brush, and the second is a = blending or crease brush to blend out hard lines.

- When blending from the crease of the eye, use very small circular motions and only use the tip of the brush, about 2–3 mm. Avoid using too much pressure.

- If the brush is separating when you are blending shadow, you are working too agressively and will create a patchy effect. Use the blending brush like feather tickling the face.

Powder Shadow Smoky Look

This fashion look, opposite, can be worked in various colour combinations, using light, mid- and dark tones of powder shadow on the eyes. Here the light tone is pale pink, the mid-tone is soft purple and the dark tones are grey and black.

1 Using a peach or nude eyeshadow, start with a neutral wash of colour applied from the eyelash line all the way up to the brow.

2 Now take a matte pale pink, the lightest colour, and apply it to the lid from the lash line to the fold of the eye using a stiff brush. Do not go any higher or you won't have space to blend out.

3 Take a soft purple, the mid-tone, and apply it from the outer corner of the eye and up over top of the crease toward the bridge of the nose, blending softly upward as you go.

4 Once you have created the correct shape, take the smoky grey and deepen the crease, again using a stiff brush.

5 Using the same brush with the darkest tone, here black, bring some of the colour underneath the eye, below the bottom lashes. This colour can be placed from the outer corner of the eye right to the inner corner.

6 Next, take a softer brush with a bit of mid-tone colour on it and blend the shadow along the lower lashes downward, softening any hard edges.

7 Using a light, shimmery shadow with a satin finish (in the same tones you have been using) and a soft brush, add a bit of highlight to the inner corner of the eye and right underneath the brow. This will brighten, lift and open up the eye.

8 Now, add black gel liner to the top lid using an angle brush and line the lower waterline with a black kohl pencil to deepen the look.

9 To finish, apply a generous amount of black mascara to the top and lower lashes.

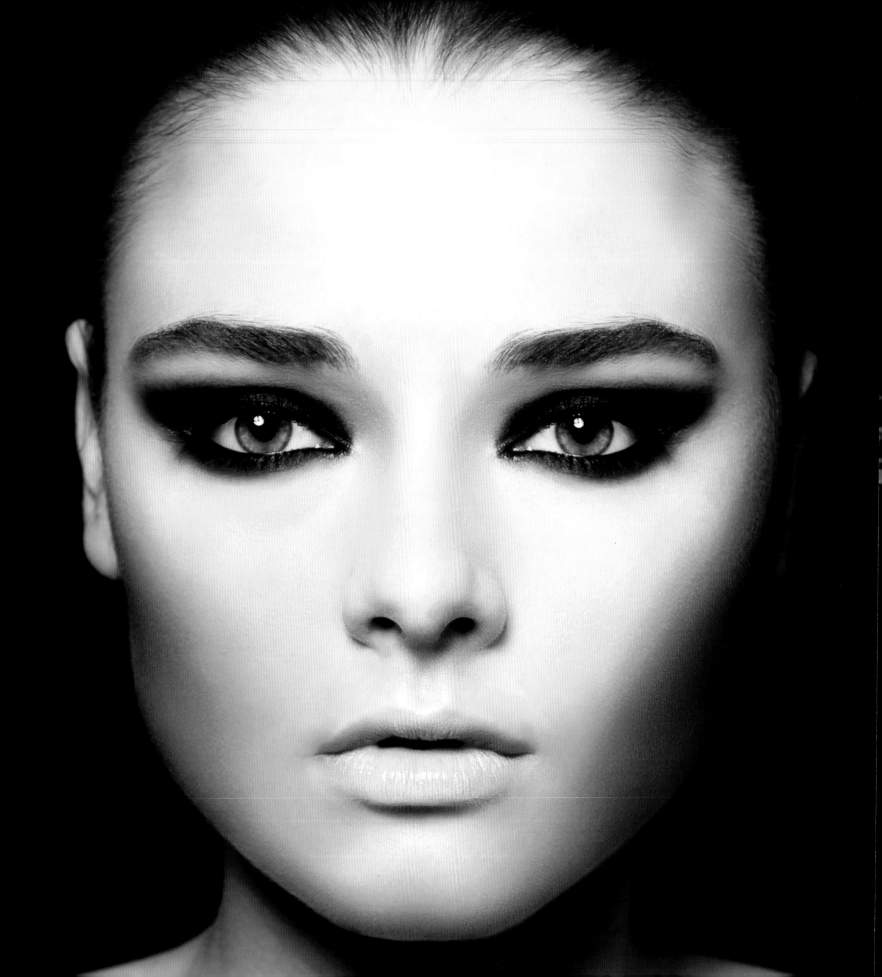

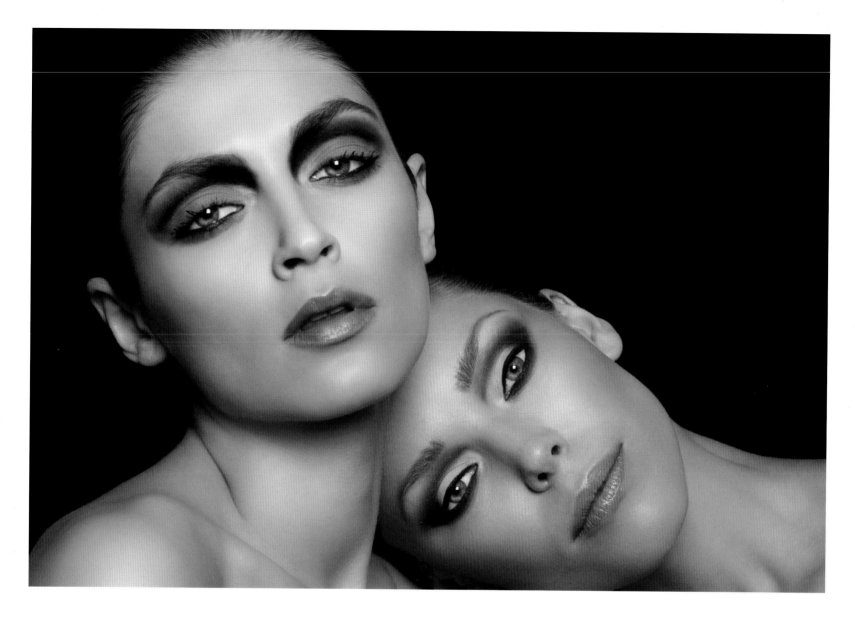

(above)
Photographer: Lou Denim **Makeup:** Jana Ririnui and Jade Hunka using MAC **Models:** Natalia Gal @ Models 1 (left) and Viktorija Skyte @ Storm (right)

(left) **Photographer:** Catherine Harbour **Makeup:** Jana Ririnui using Bobbi Brown **Model:** Jodie @ Nevs

Greasepaint Smoky Eyes

The deep, glossy look, opposite, was created using black greasepaint with black powder shadow applied over the top to set the cream. Suitable for fashion work, such as editorials and fashion shows, this is not ideal if you need to get long use out of the look, as it will crease over time.

- Using pigment rather than powder shadow on top of the greasepaint or wet gel liner will give a different effect.

- Add clear lip gloss over the top to finish a smoky eye, but only apply at the last minute or the makeup will crease quickly. This effect looks great on men for editorial shots and the more you blend out the gloss, the better.

Gel Smoky Eyes

Longwear gel eyeliner, used in the images above, is a good, quick way to do a smoky eye but it will require a bit more skill. With this method you need to work fast as the gel dries quickly, and once it has, can be tricky to blend or correct. Make sure you apply it to one eye at a time and only to one section at a time as you work.

First apply the gel eyeliner to the upper lid from the lashline to the fold of the socket. Wait until the glossy texture has dried, usually in about 2–3 minutes. Don't blend any shadow over the top until the gel is dry or you will have an uneven result.

Use the tip of a crease brush to blend and don't apply too much pressure. You can add black kohl on the inner rim of the eye and soften with black shadow under the lower lash line.

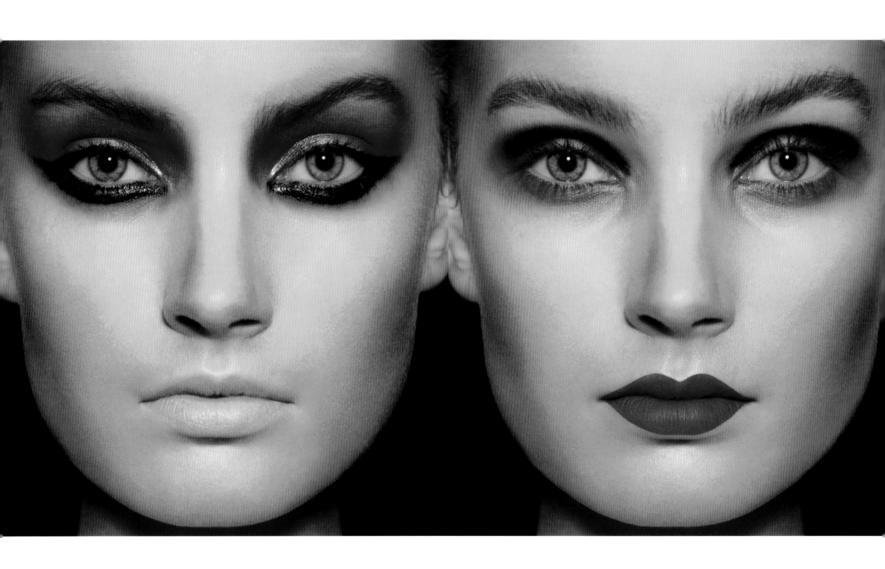

Electric Nude

Contour the upper eyelids with warm bronze tones and use an electric blue khol pencil to extend the bottom eyeliner. Striking and simply simple!

Romantic Goth

Using red and vibrant pink under the eye and on the eyelid can make the eyes look tired and severe, but adding a matte black eyeshadow into the crease of the eye – combined with velvety red lips – creates a sophisticated, romantic goth look.

Photographer: Lou
Denim **Makeup:** Jose
Bass **Model:** Joanna
Stubbs @ Models 1

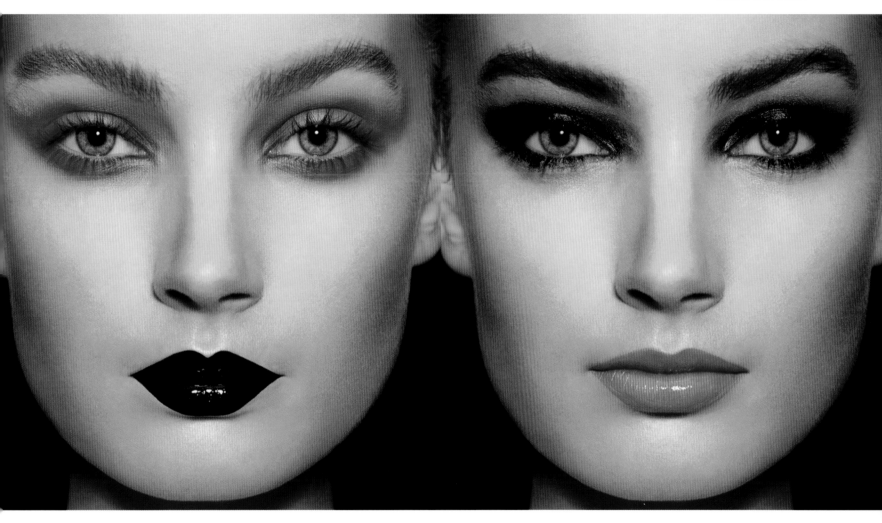

Radical Vamp

Brighten black lips by pairing them with pinks and purples. Blend the colours upward and outward, starting with lavender in the inner corners brushed up into the brows and bleeding into red and pink. If you are daring, add lime green as a brow highlight. No mascara is necessary with the black lips.

Pussycat Doll

First apply green shadow on top and blue below. For feline definition, extend black cream eyeliner on the outer edge of the eye and blend it into the crease with plenty of mascara and black khol on the upper and lower rims.

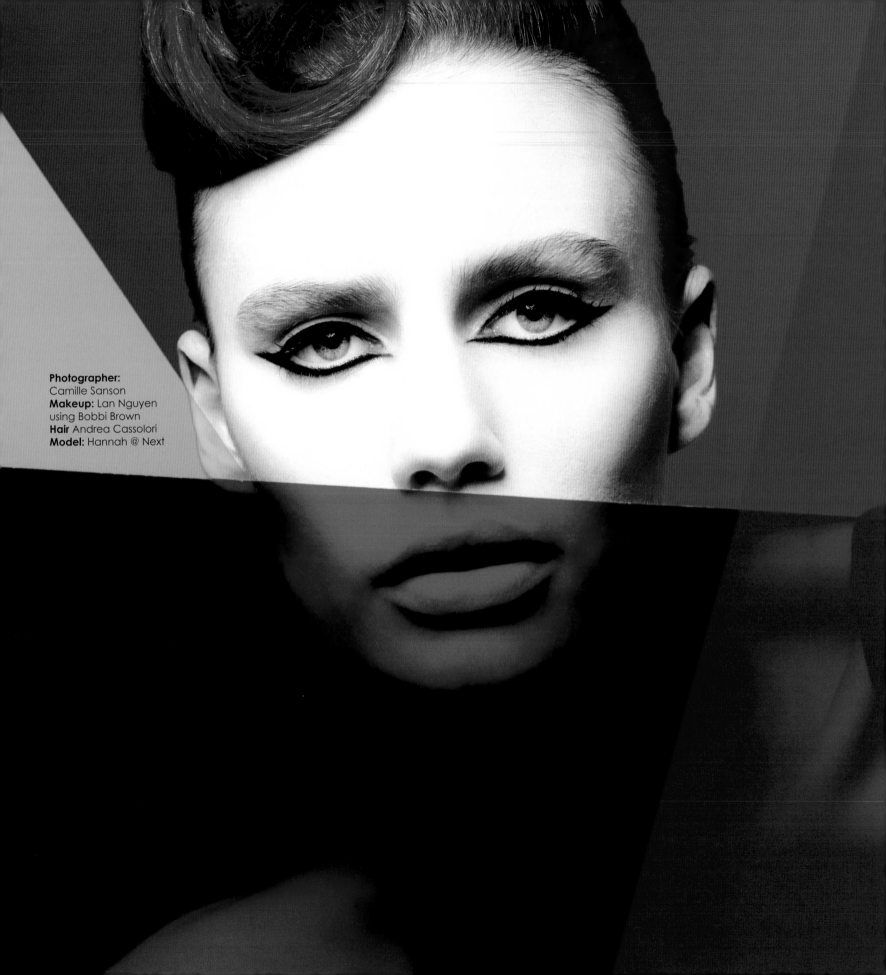

Photographer:
Camille Sanson
Makeup: Lan Nguyen
using Bobbi Brown
Hair Andrea Cassolori
Model: Hannah @ Next

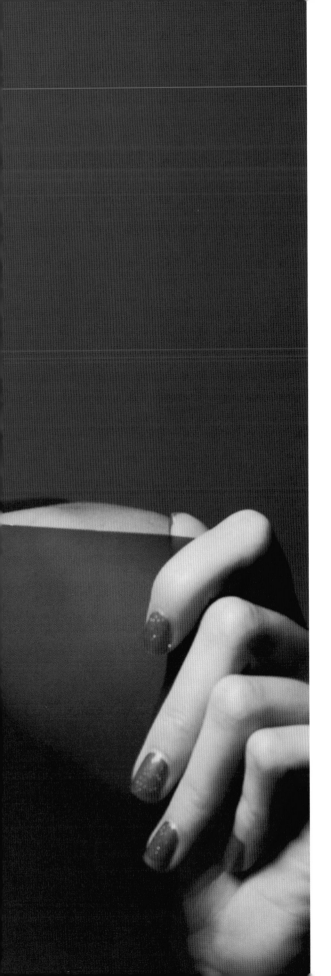

The pencil is one of the most popular forms of eyeliner. There is a huge choice, as they are available in every colour of the rainbow and in metallic, matte and satin finishes. Pencils are generally the easiest type of eyeliner to apply and, when sharpened, produce a nice clean line that is easy to correct. A common trend with makeup companies today is to produce kohl pencils with softer leads that are gentle on the eye and can be smudged to create a more smoky effect.

Using a black pencil in the inner rim of the eye will make it appear smaller and more sultry. A white pencil in the inner rim opens up the eyes, reduces the appearance of redness and makes eyes appear more bright and alert. Waterproof eyeliners should not be used on the inner rim of the eyes.

Liquid Eyeliners

A wet, almost ink-like liner, these can be applied using a brush or often come packaged with a wand or soft, pen-like nib. They range in size, from very thin brushes that create fine lines to thicker, wider brushes that create a more striking, eyeliner effect. Liquid eyeliners can take a minute or so to dry and any movement while wet can cause them to smudge. They can be tricky to use and mistakes are often messy to correct but, once dry, your liner is set all day (or night). Liquid eyeliners tend to have a shiny finish once dry.

Gel Eyeliners

As the name implies, gels have a soft, gel-like texture and need a brush to apply. They dry reasonably quickly, but can also be moved or smudged. When almost dry they give an eyeshadow effect, but with more staying power. They are less messy than their liquid counterparts and by using a fine brush you can create really precise lines.

Cake Eyeliners

A flat, pressed powder, cake eyeliner is used with a wet brush to create a bold line. This can intensify the lashes or "smoky eye" look. If the pigment is not strong enough, the eyeliner will not be as striking. A thin, flat brush or angled brush is essential. Makeup artists sometimes expand on this idea to create an eyeliner using a highly pigmented powder or eyeshadow and a wet brush dipped in a mixing medium or water. This is mainly used to create more unusual colours.

MASCARAS

Ask any makeup artist and they will tell you that the quality of a mascara is largely based on its wand. The trend in recent years is to go back to the old-school 1950s-era wands. Mascaras come in a variety of formulas and colours – from the usual blacks, browns and clear to blue, green, purple, gold, silver and white.

There are mascaras that claim to lengthen, thicken, curl, or a combination of all the above. Some come with a primer, to coat the lashes before the colour is applied. This is normally to help thicken the lashes. Then there are the new formulations of mascara, which form tubes over individual lashes, which can be removed by wiping off with water. Mascaras are also available in a waterproof formula, although these can be harder to remove at the end of the day. Although there are many great mascaras on the market, a good makeup artist can make most mascaras work for them using the following tips.

* Always curl the lashes.
* Make sure the mascara has not dried
  out – mascaras have a 2–3 month shelf
  life after opening.
* Apply a few coats of mascara, concentrating it
  at the base of the lashes and making sure that
  every lash has been coated.
* Use an eyelash comb to make sure there
  are no clumps.

In addition to mascara for eyelashes, there are also mascaras for brows. They are either used to slightly lighten or darken the eyebrows and have a more natural effect than filling in eyebrows with powders or pencils. They usually come in colours that match hair colour, such as blonde, brown, dark brown and red. Clear mascara can be used to comb and hold eyebrows in place.

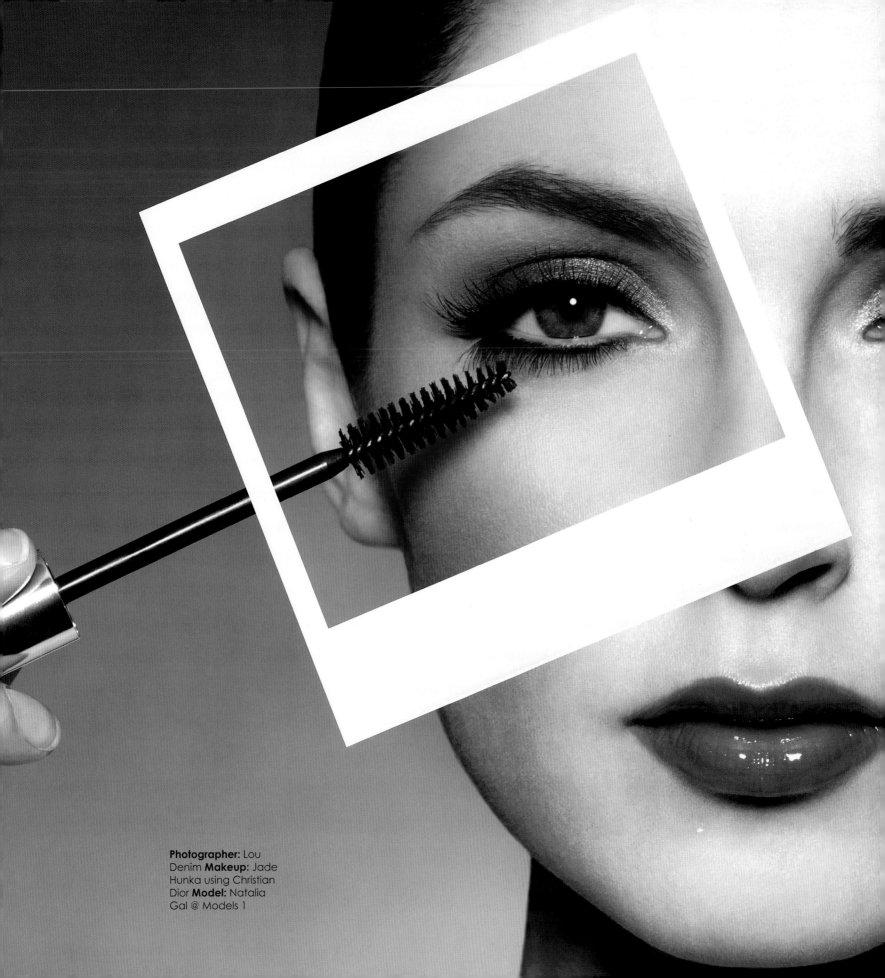

Photographer: Lou Denim **Makeup:** Jade Hunka using Christian Dior **Model:** Natalia Gal @ Models 1

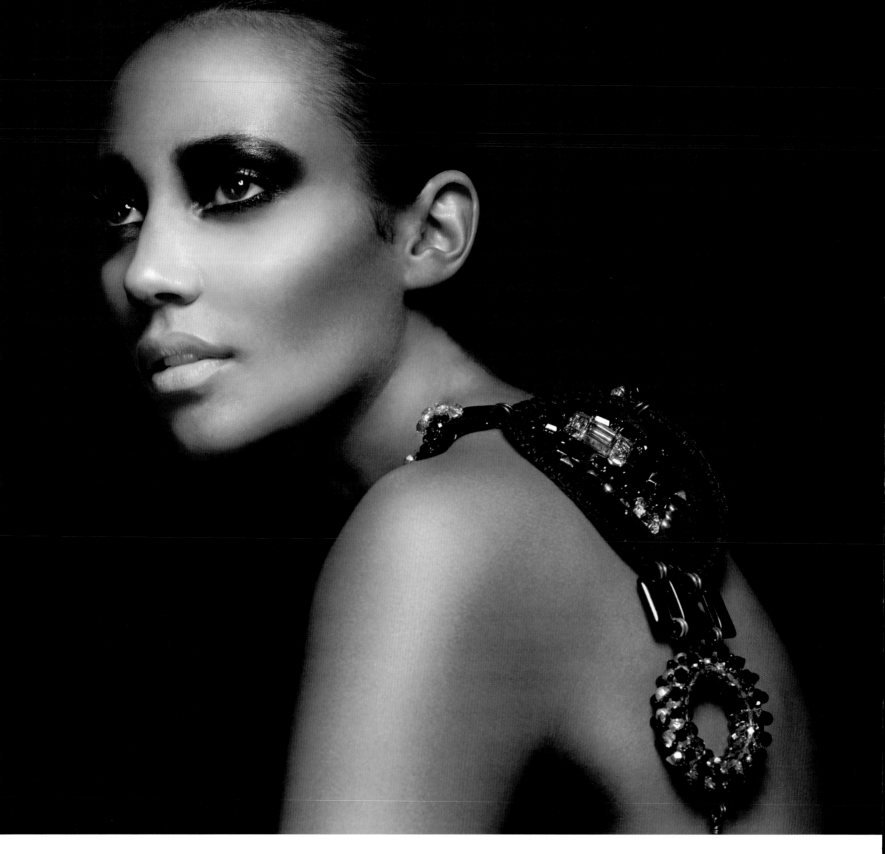

Photographer:
Catherine Harbour
Makeup: Sandra
Cooke using MAC
Hair: Nathalie Malbert
Model: Robyn @ FM

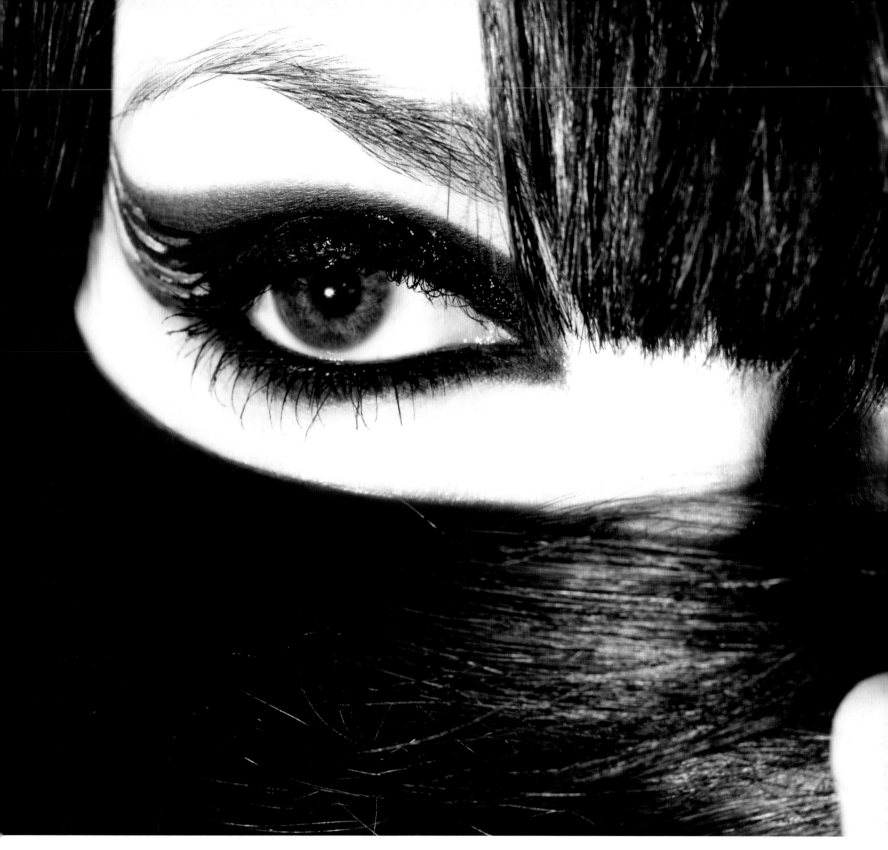

Photographer:
Camille Sanson **Hair
and Makeup:** Cristina
Iravedra using Bobbi
Brown **Model:** Claudia
@ Nevs

65

EYELASHES

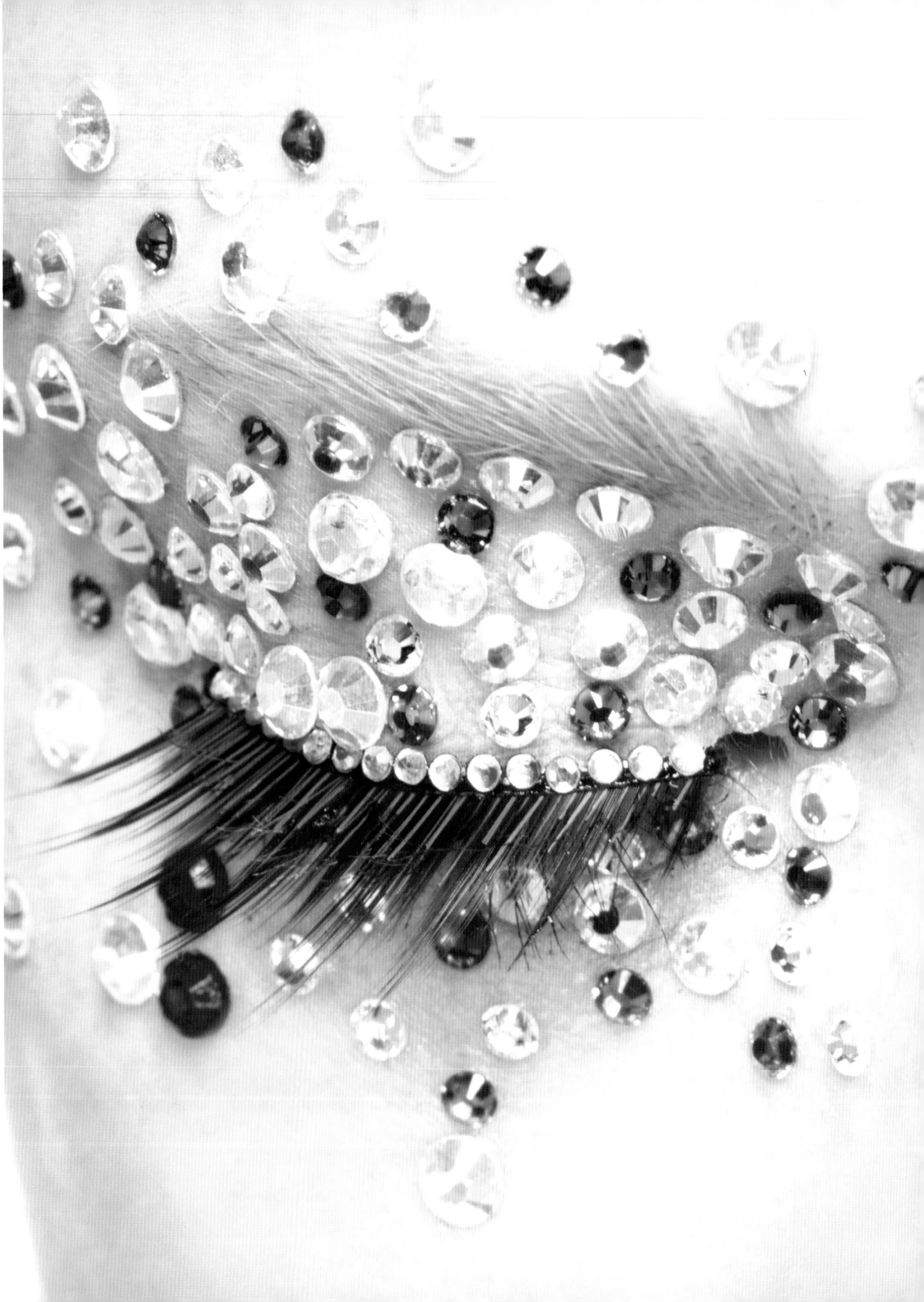

Photographer:
Keith Clouston
Makeup: Sandra
Cooke using Swarovski
Model: Michelle Easter
@ Red Models

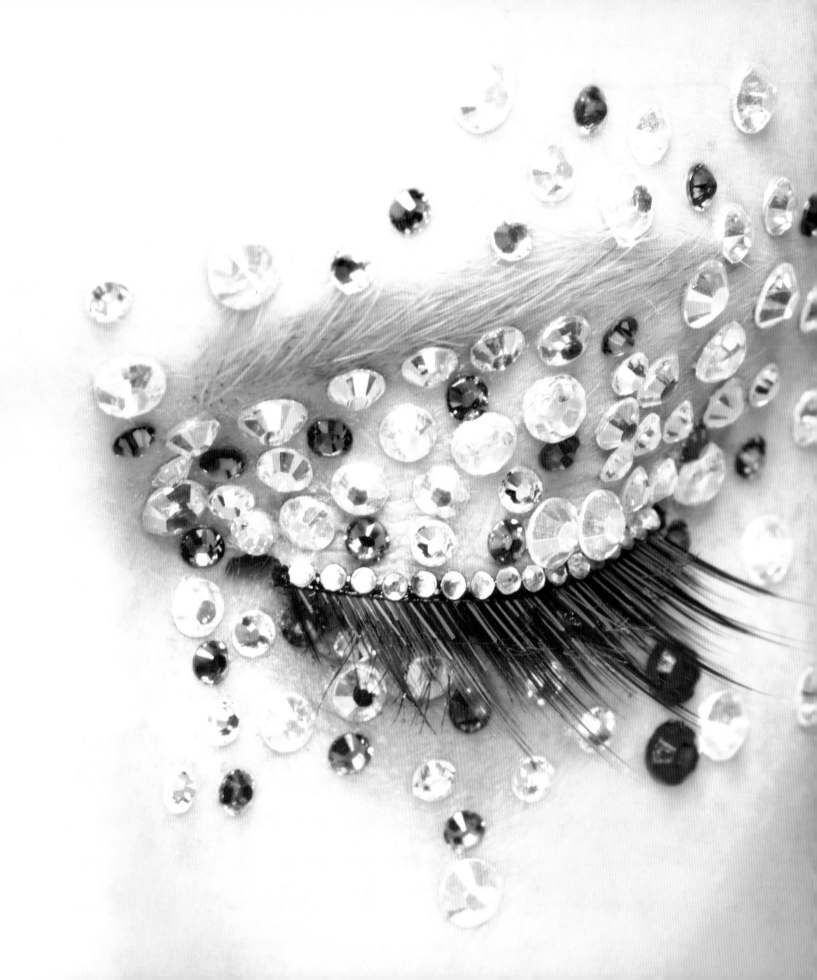

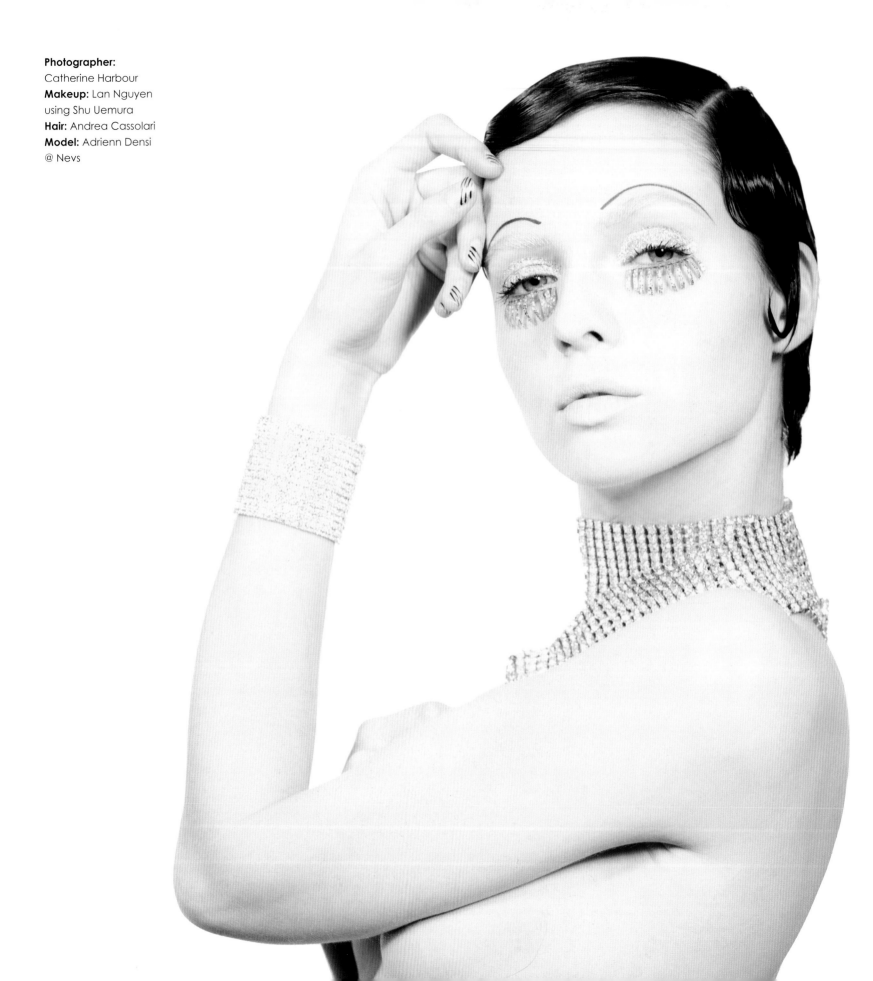

Photographer:
Catherine Harbour
Makeup: Lan Nguyen
using Shu Uemura
Hair: Andrea Cassolari
Model: Adrienn Densi
@ Nevs

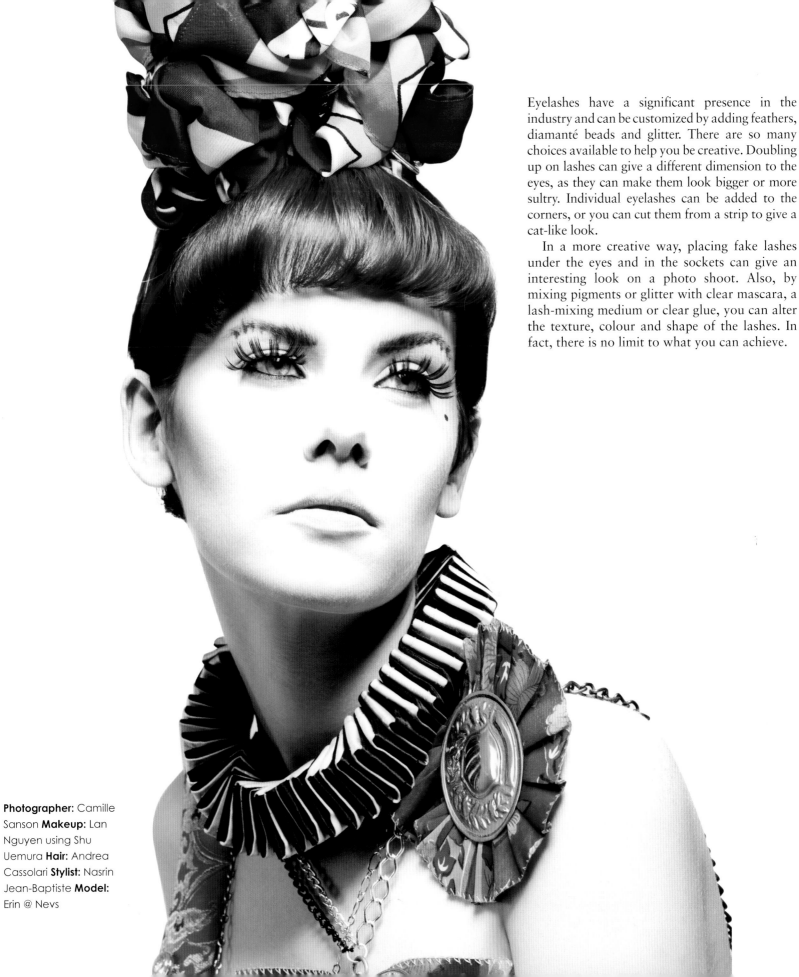

Eyelashes have a significant presence in the industry and can be customized by adding feathers, diamanté beads and glitter. There are so many choices available to help you be creative. Doubling up on lashes can give a different dimension to the eyes, as they can make them look bigger or more sultry. Individual eyelashes can be added to the corners, or you can cut them from a strip to give a cat-like look.

In a more creative way, placing fake lashes under the eyes and in the sockets can give an interesting look on a photo shoot. Also, by mixing pigments or glitter with clear mascara, a lash-mixing medium or clear glue, you can alter the texture, colour and shape of the lashes. In fact, there is no limit to what you can achieve.

Photographer: Camille Sanson **Makeup:** Lan Nguyen using Shu Uemura **Hair:** Andrea Cassolari **Stylist:** Nasrin Jean-Baptiste **Model:** Erin @ Nevs

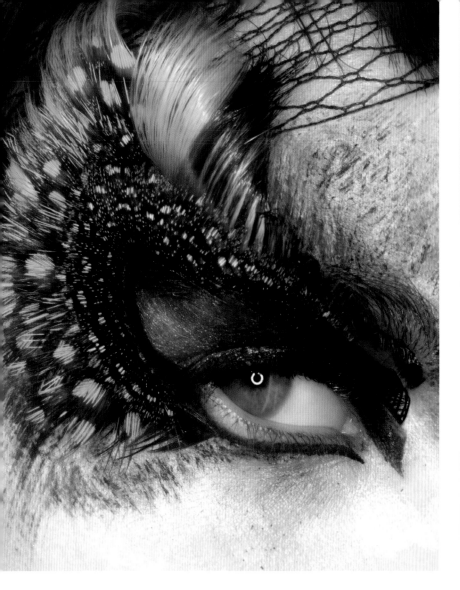

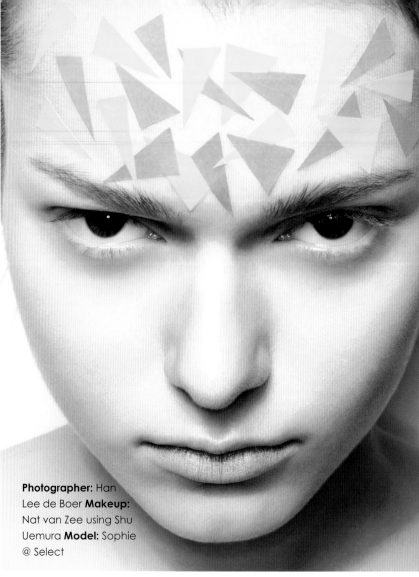

Photographer: Han Lee de Boer **Makeup:** Nat van Zee using Shu Uemura **Model:** Sophie @ Select

Green Feather Lashes

1 Using a stiff fan-shaped brush, create random brushmarks with white and black cream eyeshadow on the cheek and forehead.

2 Using black cream eyeshadow, paint an outline of a wing shape from the inner corner of the eye outward along the top lash line, and back toward the inner corner under the lower lash line. Leave a similar, minimized area on the moving part of the eyelid clear, creating a wing shape inside the larger wing shape.

3 Fill in the outer wing shape with the black cream eyeshadow and the inner wing shape with a dark green liquid makeup, such as Aquarelle Makeup Forever. Allow to dry.

4 Cover the outline of the black wing shape with various-sized feather lashes, such as those from Shu Uemura, sticking them on with eyelash adhesive. Alternatively, customize ordinary false lashes with real feathers or paper cut-outs – the more you experiment, the more individual the look can be.

Sticker Effect

The effect seen above is created by first using liquid foundation and beige contouring for the base, as in step one of the Rainbow Lash, opposite. Eyebrows are groomed with a brow gel, and neon stickers are cut into random sizes of triangles and arranged on the forehead.

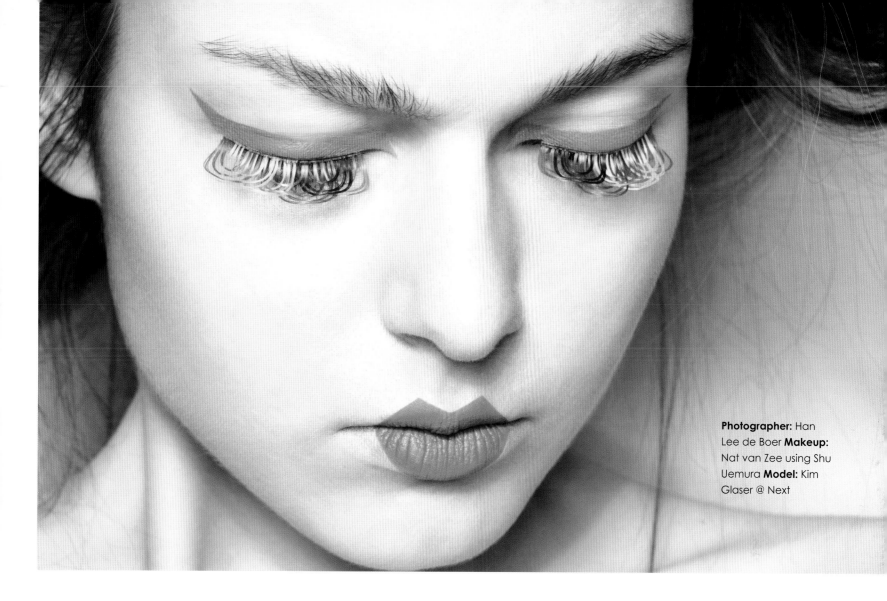

Photographer: Han Lee de Boer **Makeup:** Nat van Zee using Shu Uemura **Model:** Kim Glaser @ Next

Rainbow Lashes

1 For the base, brush a liquid foundation all over the face, and use a beige contouring powder such as MAC Sculpt & Shape in bone beige. Contour along the cheekbones to the ear and around the sides of the neck. Highlight the nose and contour along the sides of the nose.

2 Using a bright orange cream eyeshadow, line the top lashes of the eyes to create an angle at the inner corner, sloping upward at the outside corner. Build up the colour to a thick line.

3 Now glue rainbow lashes close to the top lash line. Spread the glue evenly along the edge of the lashes and let them part-dry. Then press in place gently, especially at the inner and outer edges, to get the closest fit possible.

4 For the lips, cover the outer corners with concealer and use a turquoise gel liner to create rosebud lips with an angled cupid's bow. For a perfect lip line, use a small, straight, angled brush and draw using a dot-to-dot motion with your brush as the guide line. Concealer can hide any mistakes. You can also stretch the skin taut, which will allow you to draw a clean line without gaps or bumps.

• If you find it difficult to get false lashes close enough to the natural lash line, fill in the gap with an eyeliner or eyeshadow and blend to hide the join.

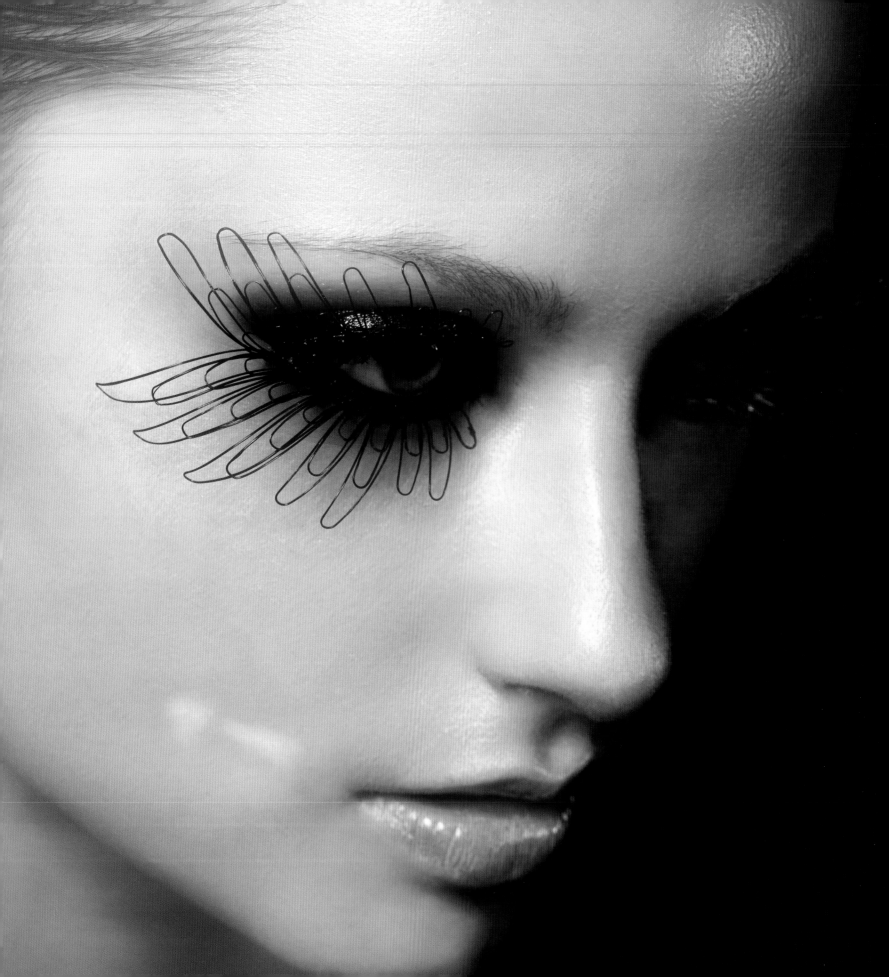

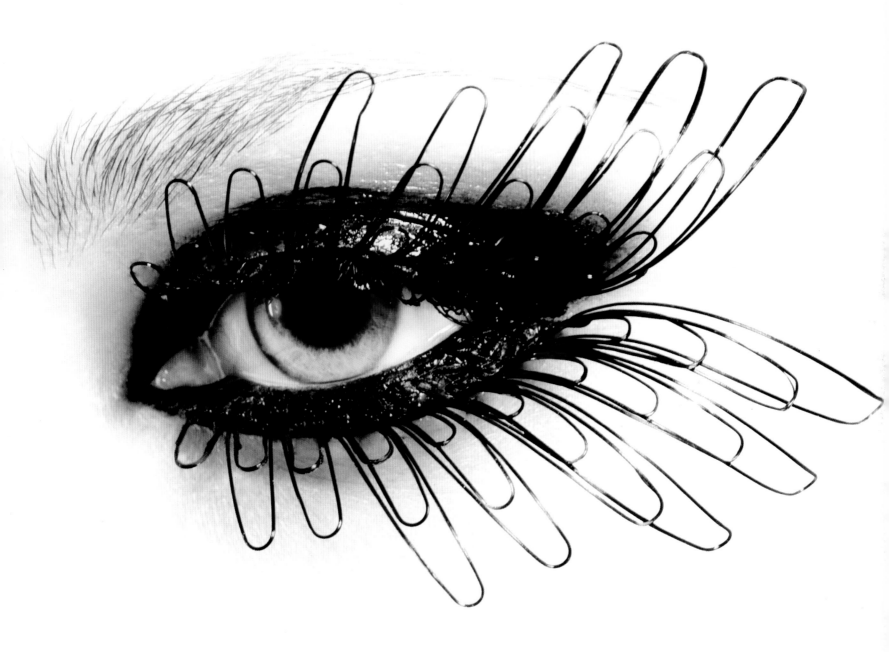

Photographer:
Catherine Harbour
Makeup: Jana Ririnui
using Shu Uemura
Model: Kasia @ First

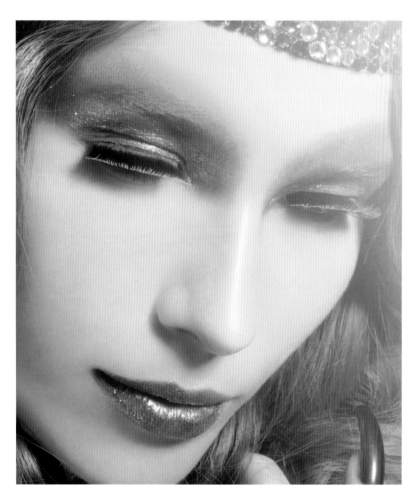 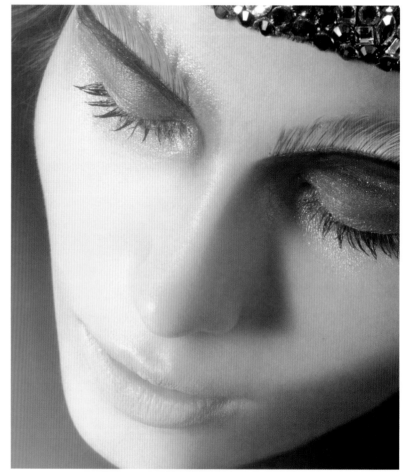

Photographer:
Fabrice Lachant
Makeup: Lan Nguyen
using Shu Uemura
Hair and skullcaps:
Marc Eastlake
Model: Monika R
@ Next

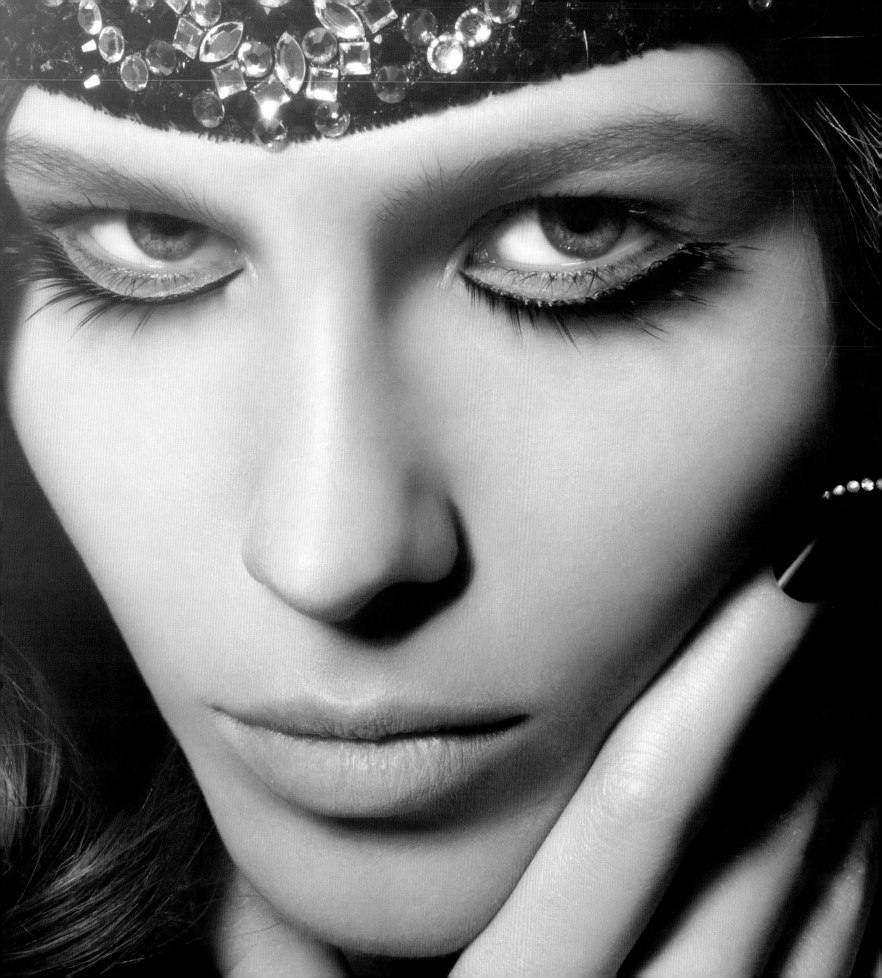

THE *LIPS*

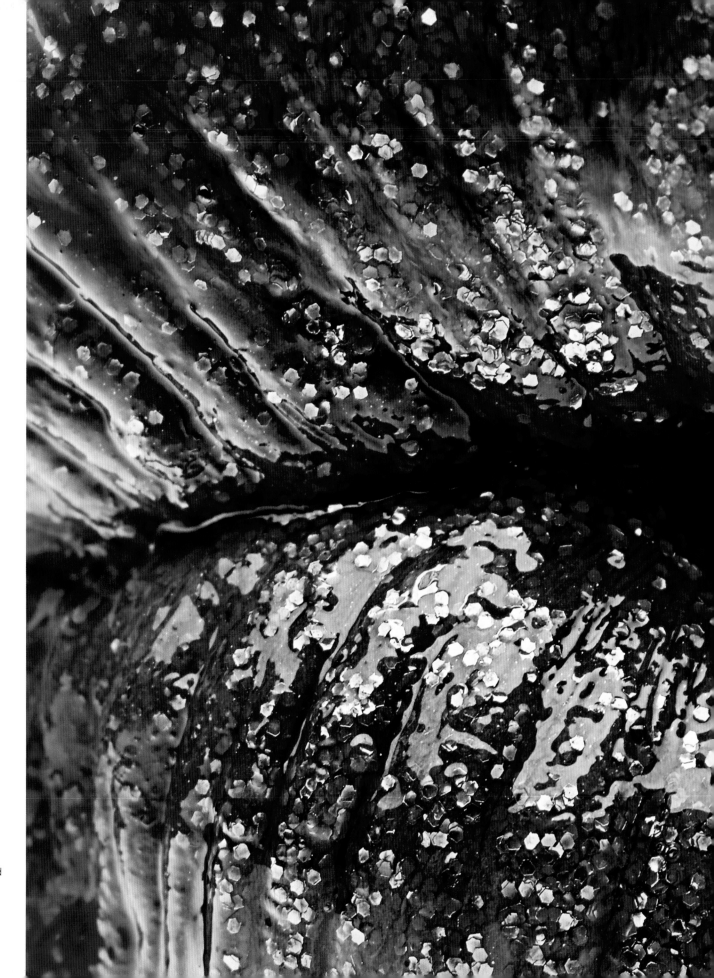

Photographer: Conrad Atton **Makeup:** Lan Nguyen using MAC

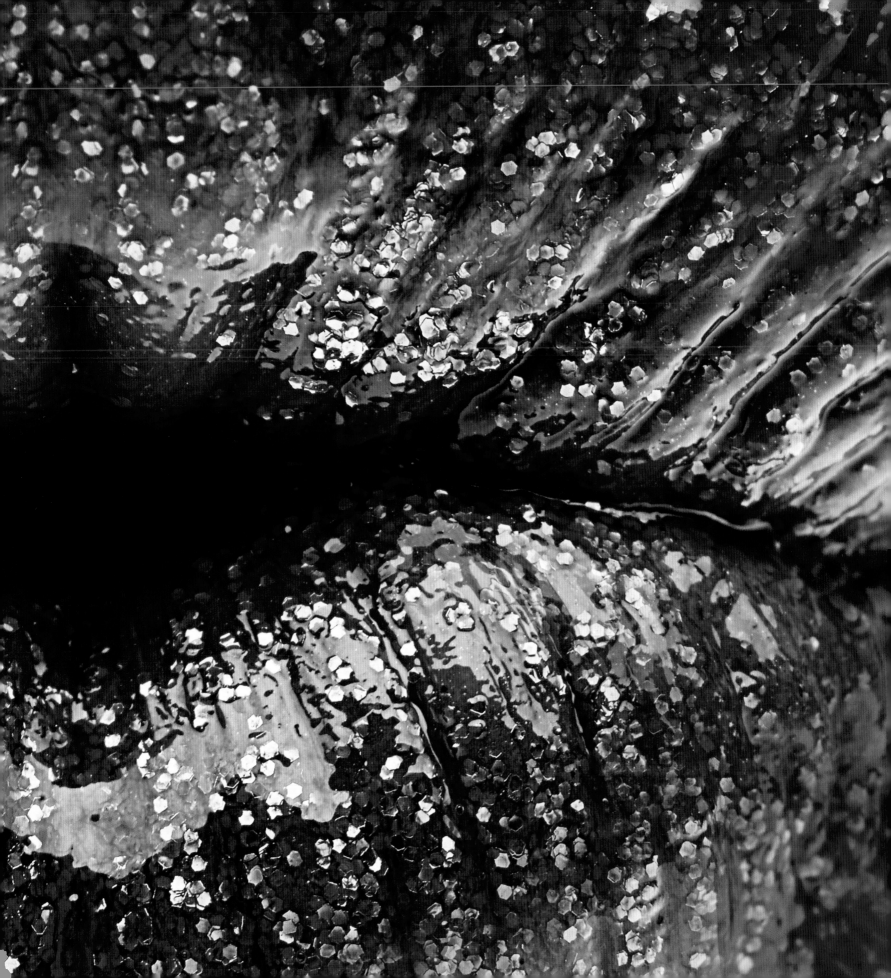

When choosing a lipstick (and this rule applies to most makeup), remember that what a product looks like in it is packaging is not always how it appears on the skin. This is because of the product's texture. In fashion and styling, makeup textures are as important as the colour.

To get a true sense of a lipstick colour, neutralize the lip with a concealer or lip primer. Lip Plump by Benefit or Lip Erase by MAC are both makeup artist favourites. Beware of cold sores on the lip area – using a lip brush on an infected area and then touching the lipstick with the brush can infect your product. Disposable lip wands, like those available from the Pro Makeup Shop (www.thepromakeupshop.com), are essential.

Preparing the Lips

It is important to prep the lip before applying lipstick, just as you would prep the skin before applying makeup to the face. Dry, flaky or cracked lips can ruin the finished result. You can gently exfoliate the lips using a treatment like Hollywood Lip's Sweet Sugar Scrub, then apply their Soothing Day Relief to heal and protect. Glam Balm by Rodial also buffs and plumps the lips.

Sheer Lipstick

This is a transparent veil of colour that allows the natural lip tone to come through by creating a see-through effect. No matter how much product you apply to the lips when using a sheer tone, the effect will be very limited in colour. Although sheers are not the best choice if you want to build a strong colour, they are a great choice when you want to create a natural makeup look with only a hint of colour. A popular example of a natural-looking sheer lipstick is Laura Mercier's Bare Lips, which is a pinky brown shade. A lip stain like Benefit's Benetint goes one step further as it colours the lips without having a coating.

Matte Lipstick

Matte lipstick gives a flat colour without shine or gloss, and most are dense in colour. As they are less likely to bleed into the fine lines around the lip area, they are great for more mature models. Matte lipsticks are also good for creating period looks from the 1920s to the 1950s (see pages 96–103). For example, if you wanted to create a 1940s lip, a matte red like MAC's Russian Red would be perfect.

Cream or Satin Lipstick

Lipsticks that are cream- or satin-textured have a smooth appearance with a touch of sheen that appears almost moist. Cream and satin lipsticks can have different levels of transparency depending on the brand. They are a good choice for bridal makeup, as they have a hint of moisture and more colour than a sheer lipstick. Ladies Choice lipstick by Benefit is a pert-toned pink with a satin/cream texture that is perfect for brides.

Frost Lipstick

Frosted lipsticks have a touch of glimmer or metallic added to the colour to create a shimmer effect. Frosted lipsticks can also have different variations of transparency, like cream or satin tones. They are a good choice if you want to create lips with reflective shine without using lip gloss. Revlon's Silver City Pink is a terrific choice for a 1960s retro lip.

Opaque Lipstick

Opaque lipstick has a dense colour and is used to fully cover the natural lips. An opaque lipstick can have a matte, satin, frost or gloss finish, but the colour is non-transparent. An example of an opaque lipstick with frost and a touch of sheen is CB96 by MAC – it is an orange lipstick that also has gold frost running through it, but the colour is full-on. If you want to create lips with high colour it is best to choose one that is opaque.

Applying Lip Colour

Always block out the lips with concealer or foundation before applying lipstick, to create a clean base – the colours will also appear truer. Lipliners are useful to recreate a different lip shape or to enhance the existing fullness. By colouring the whole lip you can build a solid base, and then add a lipstick to intensify the colour. Other products, such as eyeshadow, cream eyeshadow, loose powder pigment, greasepaints and blush creams, can also be used on the lips.

- Pressing the product onto the lips firmly with your finger is sometimes easier to control. Adding gloss on top will give volume to the lips, and by mixing colours you can create interesting tones. Using shimmer or glitter on top gives high shine for photo shoots.

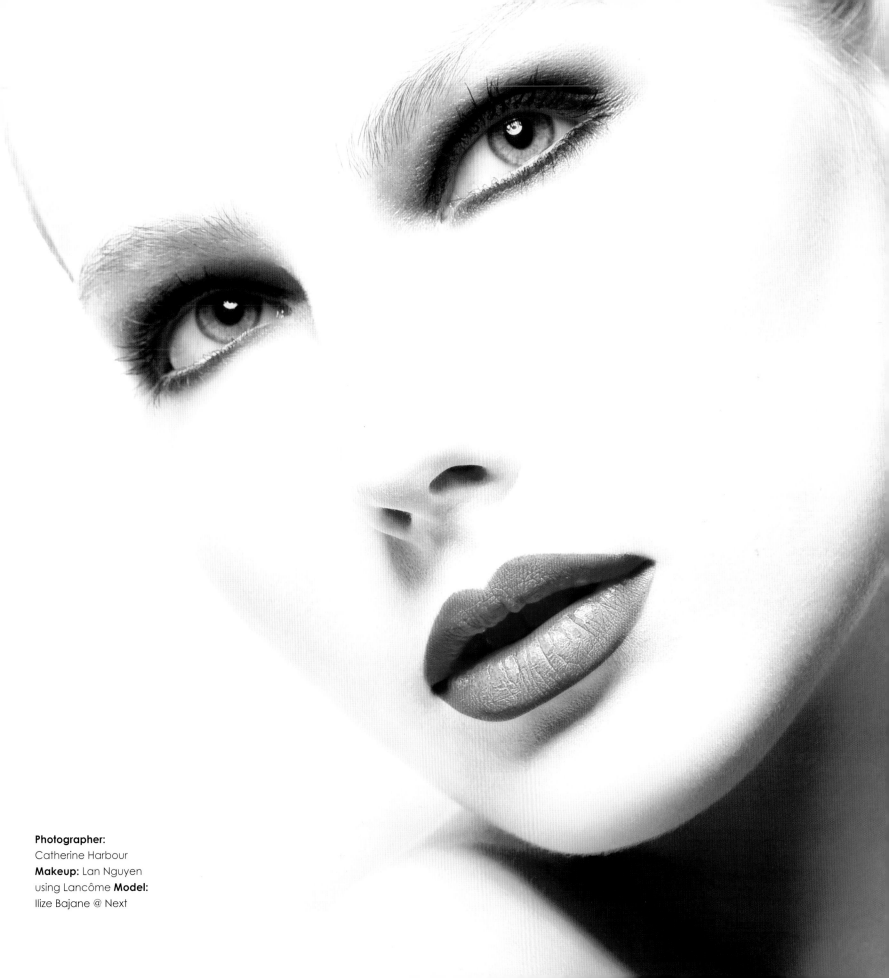

Photographer:
Catherine Harbour
Makeup: Lan Nguyen
using Lancôme **Model:**
Ilize Bajane @ Next

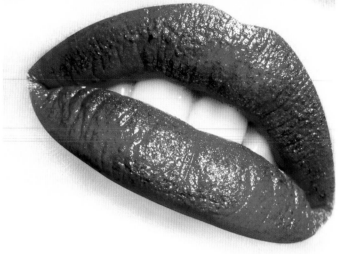

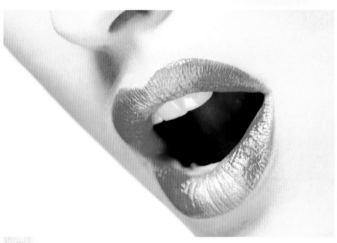

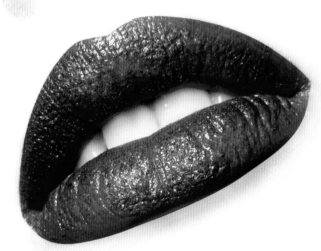

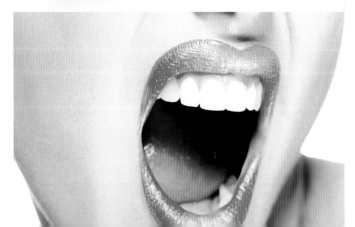

VAMPire Lips

The inspiration for vamp lips comes from Bram Stoker's 1897 novel *Drakula* and films such as *Lost Boys* (1987), *Nosferatu* (1922) and the cult classic *Vamp* (1986) starring Grace Jones.

1 Prepare the lips with a lip primer, then block out the colour with a foundation appropriate for your skin tone.

2 Choose a shade of red lipstick that suits your complexion: a blue-based red if your skin is pink-beige or a warm red if your skin is golden-beige. Apply with a lip brush for precision.

3 Line your lips top and bottom with a black pencil or black cream eyeliner. Using a lip brush, blend the black lipliner into the lipstick.

4 For more dimension dab a bit of clear lipgloss on the top and bottom middle of your lips.

Blood-Red Stained Lips

Stained lips look sophisticated, effort-less and can even appear to be something of an accident. Creating the look, however, is far from accidental!

1 Prepare by applying a lip serum for smoothness, and then a lip balm for moisturizing.

2 Choose a shade of light or dark red (preferably satin or matte, nothing glossy) that suits your skin tone. If your skin is pink-beige go for a cool red; if it is golden-beige reach for a warm red.

3 Squeeze a bit of lip balm on a mixing palette and add a few scrapes of the lipstick. Mix them together with a spatula.

4 With a lip brush or, even better, with your ring finger, take a bit of the moisturizer/lipstick mix and dab it on the pout of the lips, pushing the colour in. Concentrate the colour application on the middle of the lips and work your way to the outer corners. Keep dabbing your colour mix until your lips are fully stained.

5 With a tissue or a cotton swab go around the mouth to clean any excess product and give more of that unfinished "work in progress" look. To finish, top up with a bit more lip balm.

Bubble-Gum Lips

A bubble-gum pout is a luscious, juicy pout, inspired by the mouthwatering sensation of chewing gum and popping bubbles. Think pink and lots of gloss.

1 Prepare the lips by drenching them in lip balm. Apply a bit of concealer that is a shade or two lighter than your foundation around your mouth so the gloss, when applied, will not "bleed".

2 For staying power, line your lips with a pink lipliner. Remember to choose a cool undertone pink if your skin is pink-beige or a warm undertone pink if your skin is golden-beige.

3 Brush on a pink lipstick that is suitable for your skin, depending on whether you have a cool undertone or a warm undertone.

4 Pick three lip glosses – light, medium and dark – so you can add dimension, again choosing between cool and warm tones.

5 Apply the lightest lip gloss in the middle of your pout, the medium lip gloss from the middle to the outer corners and the dark focusing on the corners of the lips.

6 Smack your lips, and pop you go!

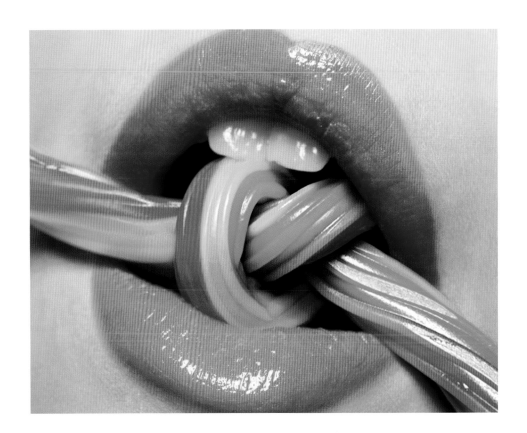

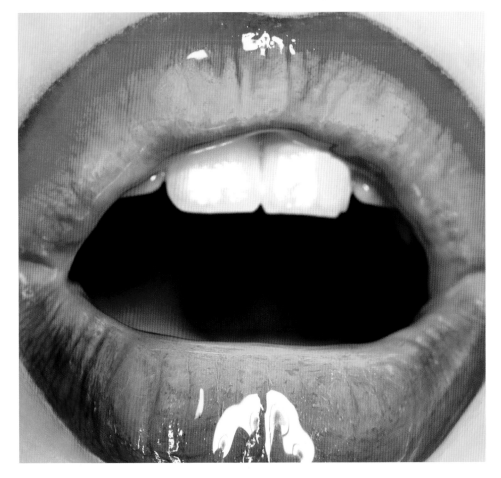

(red and purple lips, left) **Photographer:** Catherine Harbour **Makeup:** Lan Nguyen using Dior. (orange and yellow lips, left) **Photographer:** Keith Clouston **Makeup:** Sandra Cook using MAC **Model:** Lina O'Connor @ Nevs

(bubble-gum lips, top right) **Photographer:** Catherine Harbour **Makeup:** Rachel Wood using MAC. (rainbow lips, right) **Photographer:** Catherine Harbour **Makeup:** Maria Papadopoulou using MAC **Model:** Heather West @ Nevs

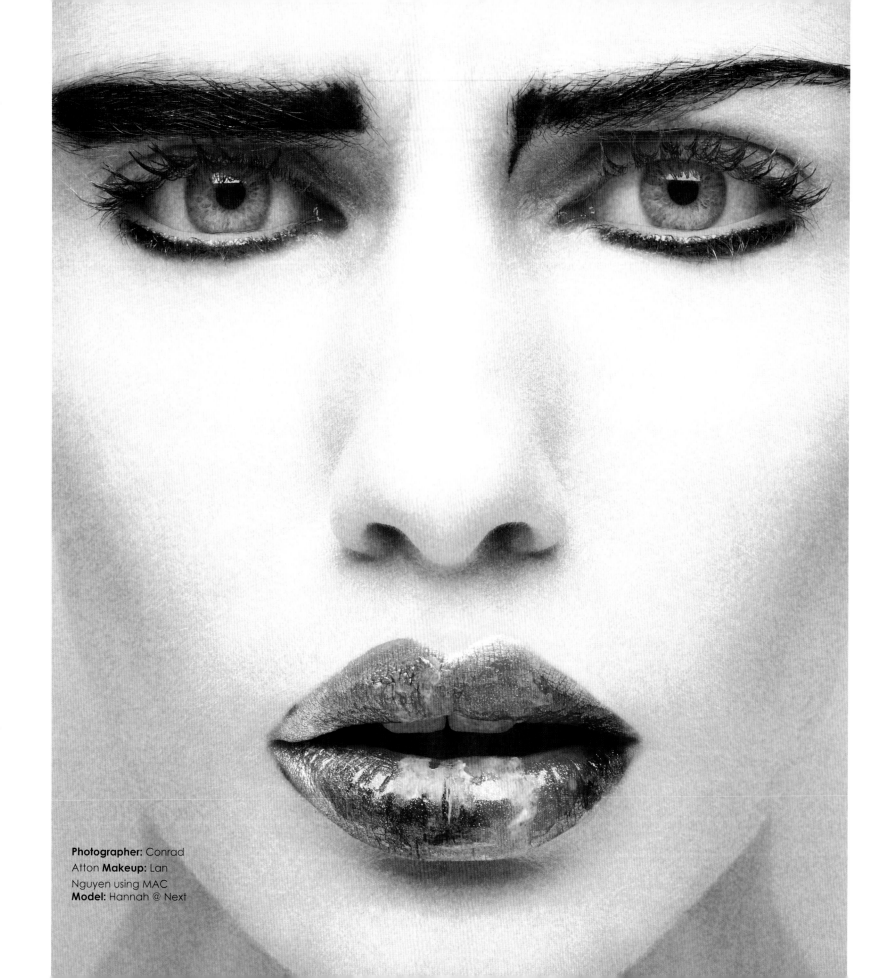

Photographer: Conrad Atton **Makeup:** Lan Nguyen using MAC
Model: Hannah @ Next

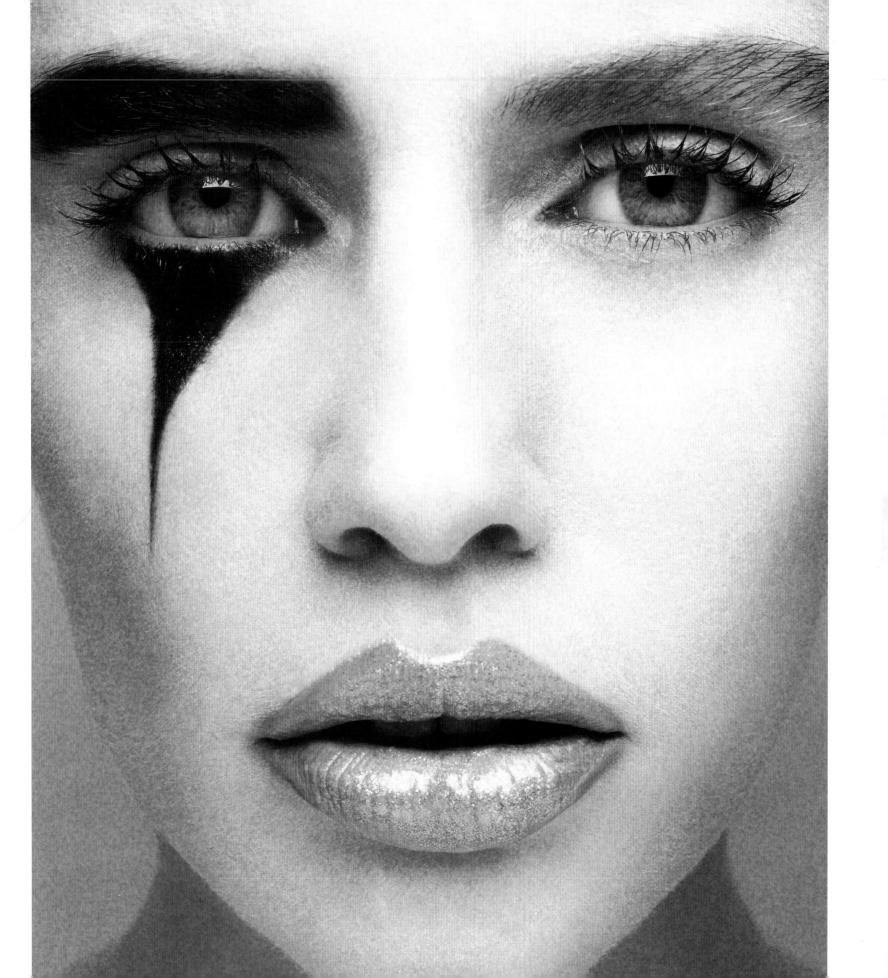

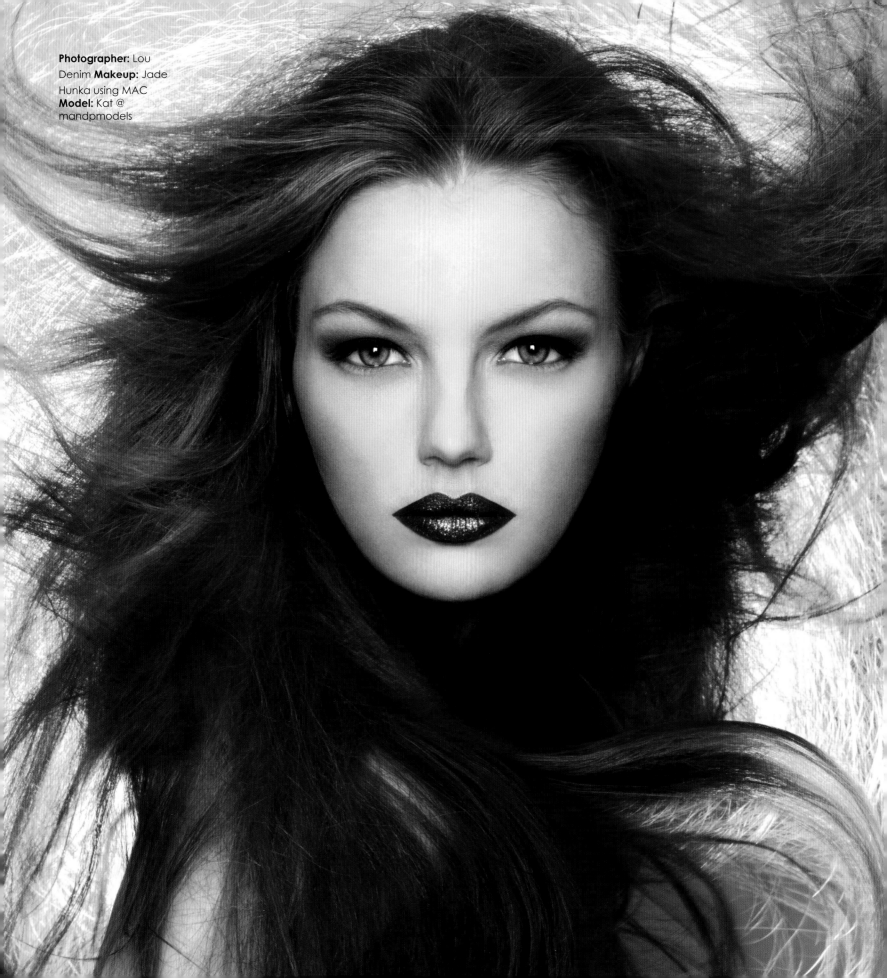

Photographer: Lou
Denim **Makeup:** Jade
Hunka using MAC
Model: Kat @
mandpmodels

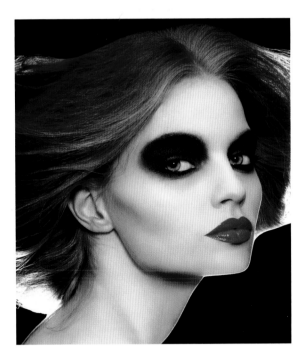

Strong Eyes and Lips

1 Apply a medium-coverage foundation to the face using a duo-fibre foundation brush and buff it into the skin for more natural, even coverage.

2 Next, apply concealer only to areas needed, using a small, synthetic brush and blending in with the fingers using a stipple/patting motion. The heat from your fingers will help push the product into the skin, while the stipple motion allows you to build coverage without moving the product outward from the area needed.

3 Powder more oily areas on the face, such as the forehead, nose and chin. Also powder underneath the eye to set the concealer and prevent it from creasing, and the lid, too, to set the foundation and create a smooth base for eyeshadow.

4 For the eyes, start off with a flat application brush and pick up some dark green shadow. Apply from the lash line up to the crease.

5 Take a soft blending brush and some mid-tone green shadow and buff the hard edge out and upward from the crease. Using two greens will give a soft gradation from dark to light, therefore creating that "smoky" look.

6 Next, take a kohl pencil in the deepest green you can find and apply generously to the top lash line. Take a stiff, round-tip brush and blend the line out to deepen the look and thicken the line.

7 Take an angle brush and a bright yellow shadow and apply colour densely and evenly directly underneath the lower lashes. You can blend the shadow out by pulling it downward to create a softer look if preferred.

8 Take a light gold/champagne shadow or other soft highlight colour and apply it to the inner corner of the eye and underneath the eyebrow. This will help lift and open up the eye.

9 Finally, apply a volumizing mascara to the top and bottom lashes and build up the intensity by increasing the amount of coats you put on.

10 Now move on to the brows. Using a clean angle brush and a shadow that matches the brows, softly fill in the hairs in a short, sweeping motion. If you apply too much product, comb through the brow using a disposable mascara wand to lift the excess colour out.

11 For the cheeks, take an angled contour brush and a cool-toned contour colour. Apply this right underneath the cheekbone, pulling from the hairline toward the nose.

12 Next, take a soft blush brush and apply a deep pinkish/red colour on the apples of the cheek, blending out on the rest of the cheekbone.

13 Highlight the top of the cheek bone by using a light-coloured shimmer and a smaller brush.

14 On the lips, use a dark purple/burgundy lip pencil to follow the natural lip line. Fill in the rest of the lips with the liner to prolong the wear of the lipstick and intensify the colour.

15 Using a synthetic lip brush and a lipstick that closely matches the lipliner colour, apply colour right up to the lip line but do not over-apply.

16 To finish the look, mix gold glitter with clear gloss and apply all over the lips. Alternatively, for a more subtle look, use a shiny, gold gloss.

Photographer: Lou Denim **Makeup:** Sharka P **Model:** Kat @ mandpmodels

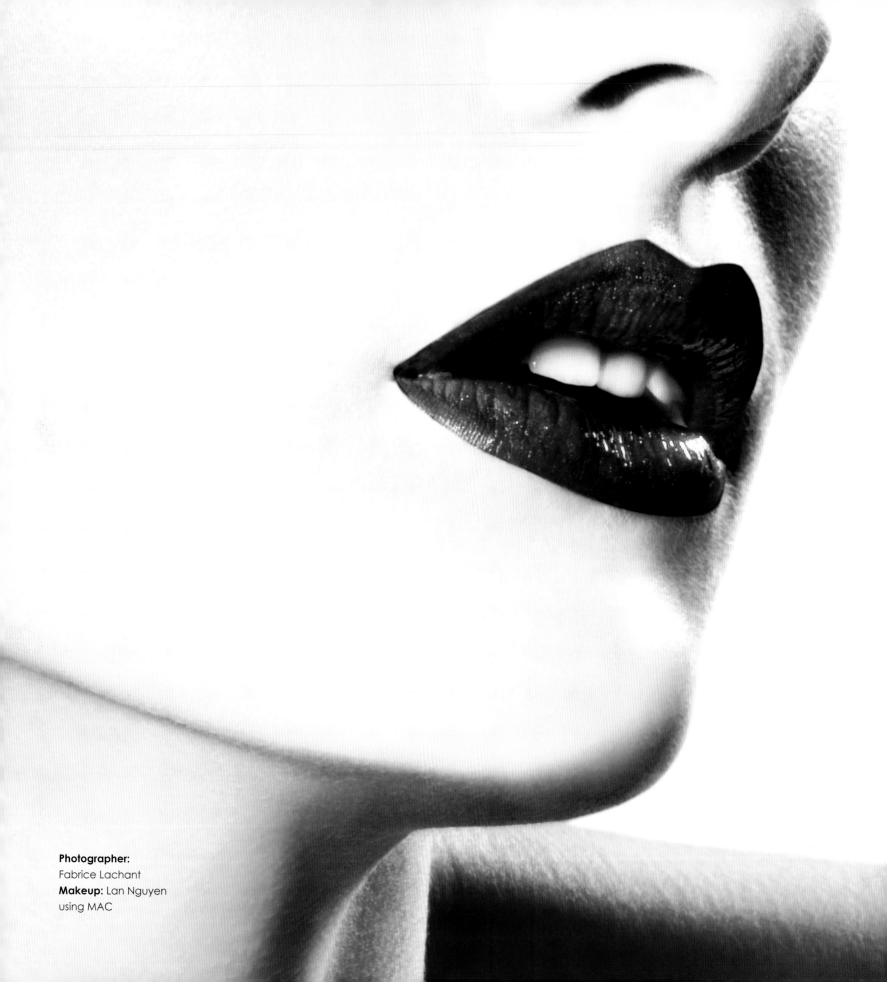

Photographer:
Fabrice Lachant
Makeup: Lan Nguyen
using MAC

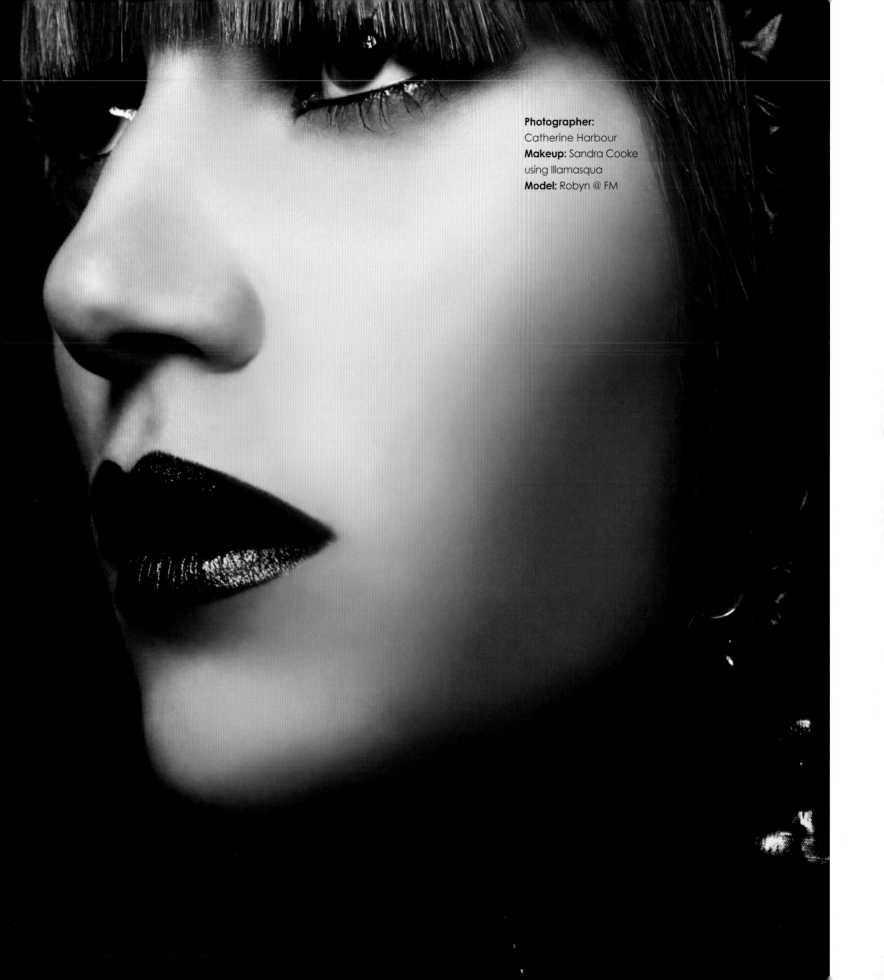

Photographer:
Catherine Harbour
Makeup: Sandra Cooke
using Illamasqua
Model: Robyn @ FM

MEN

The cosmetic industry is no longer the sole domain of women. There has been a major shift in attitudes toward men's grooming in the last decade, which has been reflected in the growing number of cosmetic ranges designed and targeted toward men. It initially started with products for shaving, and has since expanded into skincare and makeup.

"Grooming" is the term commonly used to describe hair and makeup for men at a photo shoot. The art of grooming is to make the male model look fresh, with clear skin and groomed hair, without appearing to be made up. In the days of film and soft lighting, grooming was less important, but in today's high-definition environment it is important for male models look their "natural" best.

In addition, the prominence of male models in the fashion industry is also increasing. There are more dedicated male fashion magazines (such as *GQ* and *Maxim*), men's fashion editorial stories (featuring male models and menswear designers) and also men's fashion weeks that are held in Milan and Paris each season.

Grooming generally involves cleansing and moisturizing the skin, correcting skin tone, concealing blemishes, reducing shine, combing the brows and shaving or plucking facial hair if required. If you are at a photo shoot with no stylist, then grooming also involves cutting and trimming as well as styling the hair. Grooming is not just limited to above the neck, but also includes ensuring the hands and nails are in good shape, that the body is well moisturized and the skin tone is correct.

Increasingly though, for catwalk and editorial pieces, grooming can also include applying eye makeup, such as eyeshadows and eyeliners, contouring and highlighting the face, and even applying crazy paints and colours. At men's fashion weeks, there are dedicated teams of makeup artists, hair stylists and nail technicians to groom and apply makeup for the male models to mirror the visions of the designers. So, it seems that the future of grooming will no longer be grooming only, but rather the art of makeup.

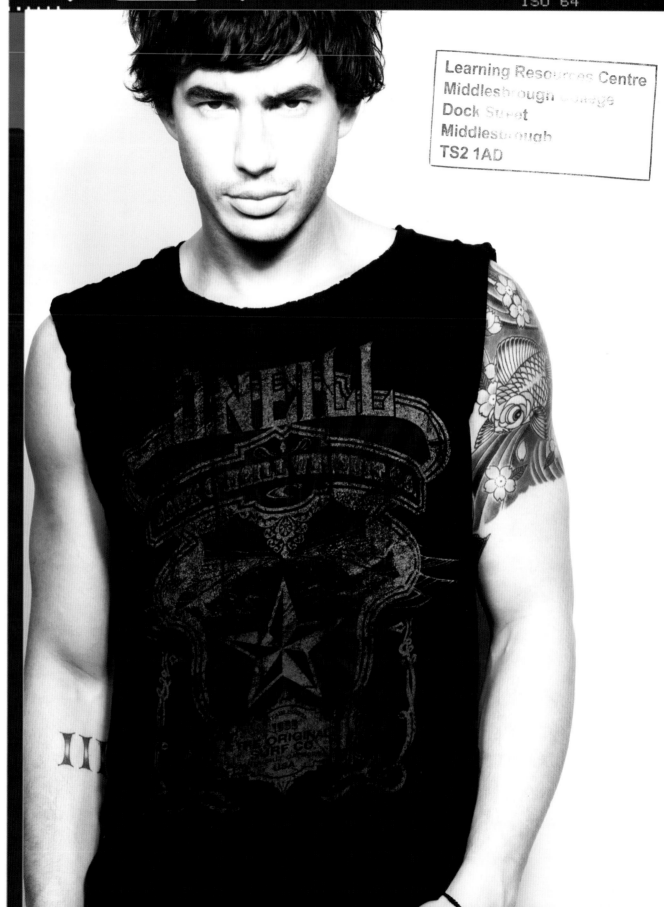

Photographer:
Catherine Harbour
Grooming: Lan Nguyen
using Kiehl's **Model:**
Nicholas Robinson

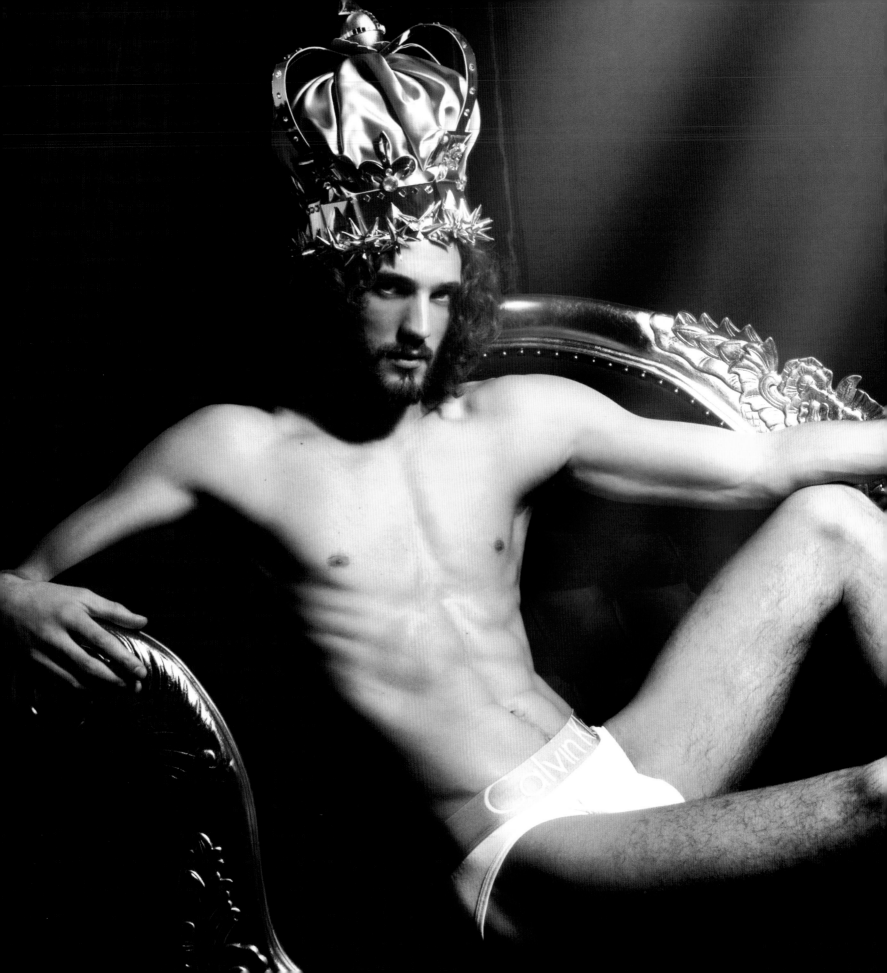

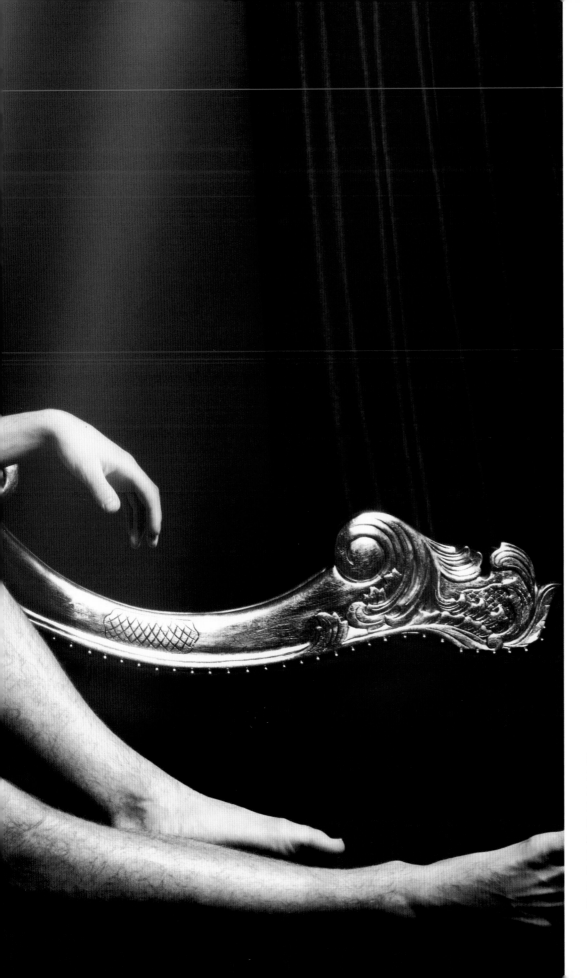

Photographer: Fabrice
Lachant **Grooming:**
Lan Nguyen using
Lancôme Homme
Stylist: Karl Willett
Model: Max @
Dynamite Hosts.
Crown by Fred
Butler, underwear
by Calvin Klein

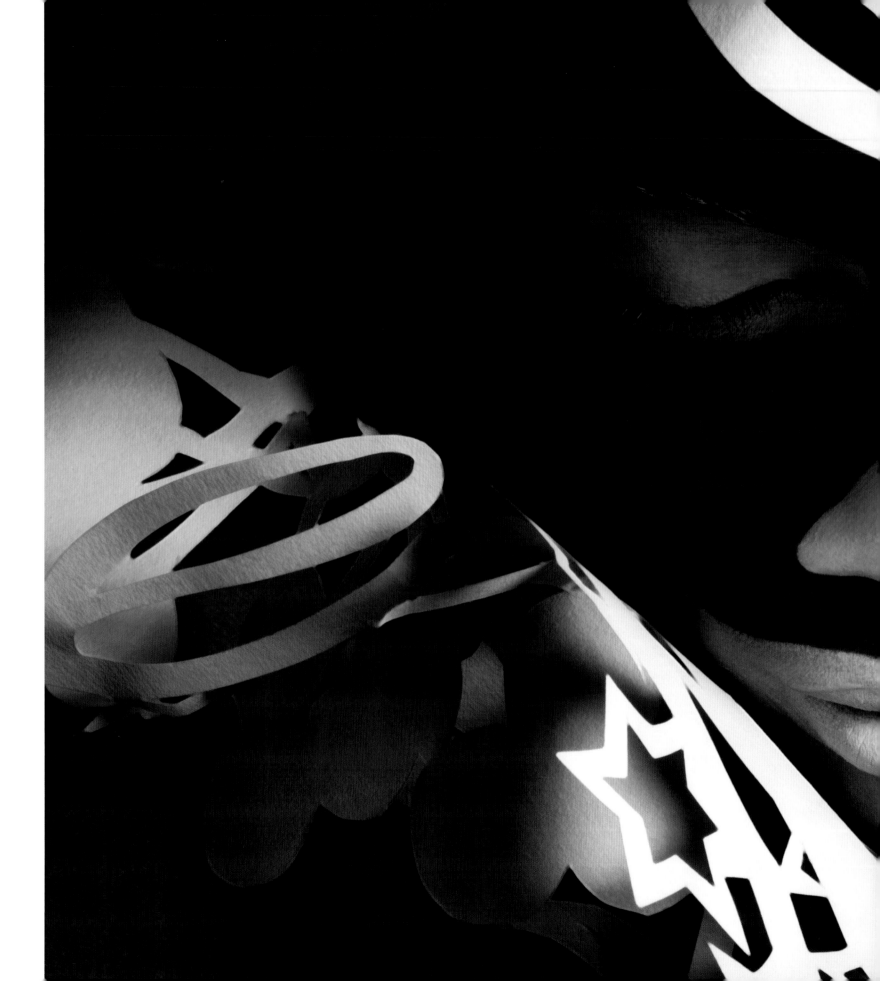

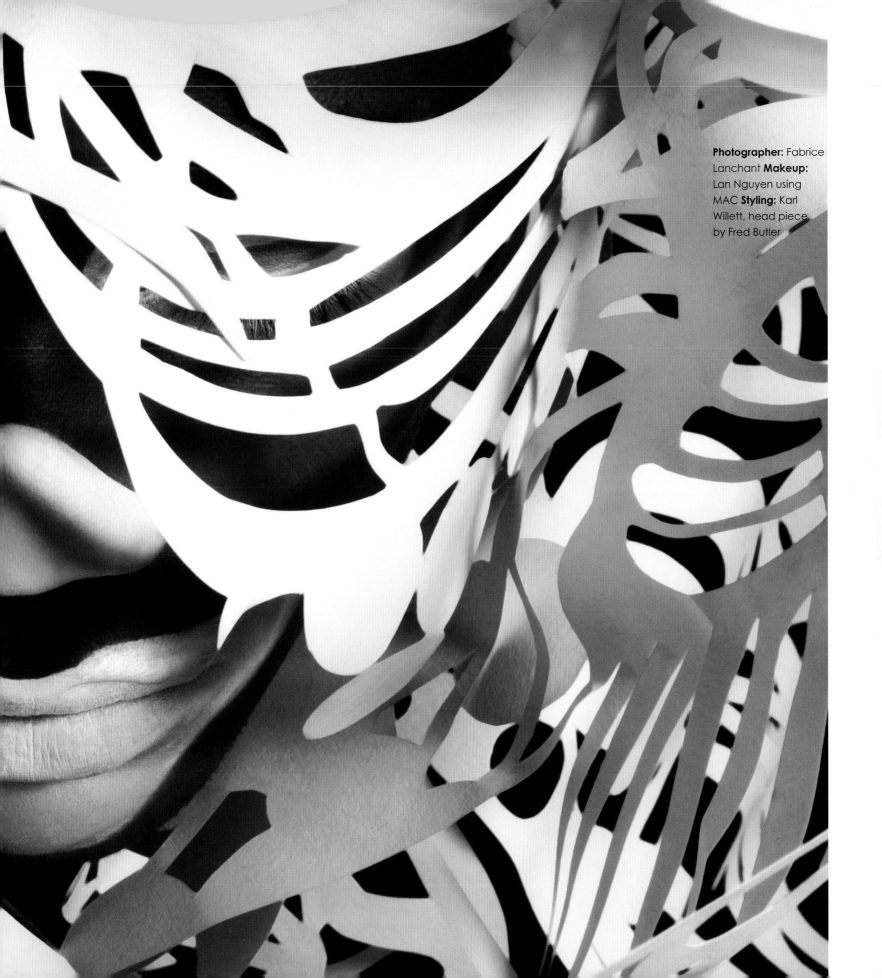

Photographer: Fabrice Lanchant **Makeup:** Lan Nguyen using MAC **Styling:** Karl Willett, head piece by Fred Butler

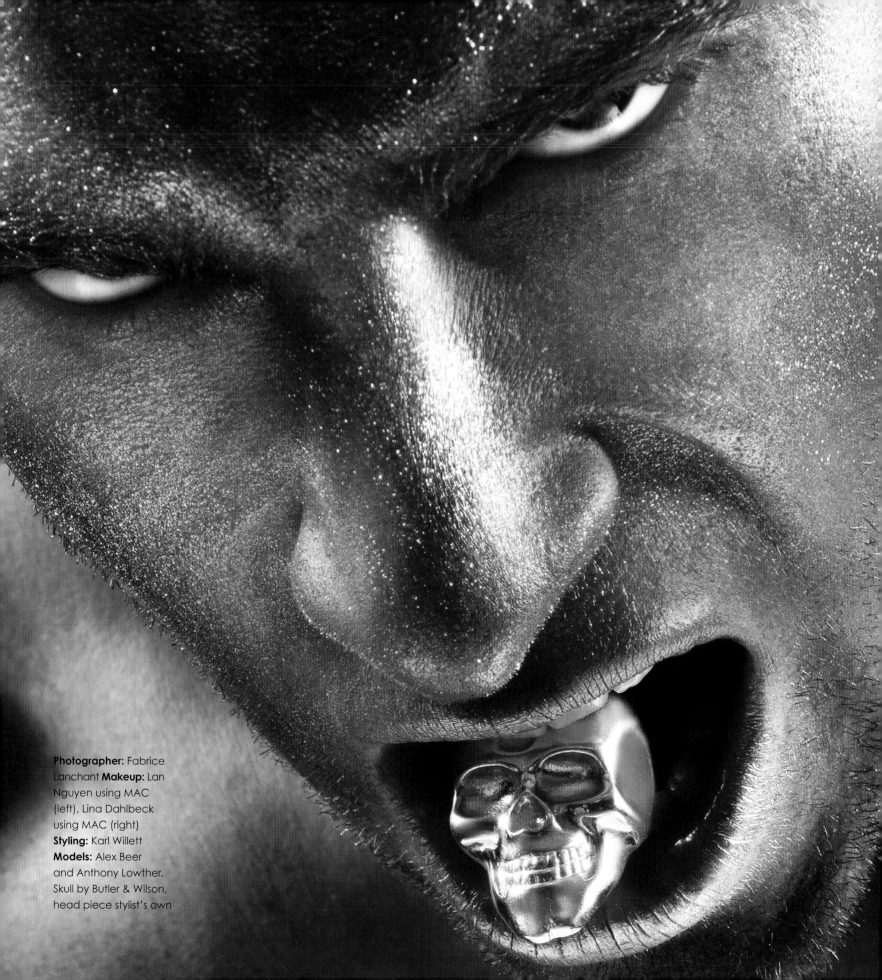

Photographer: Fabrice Lanchant **Makeup:** Lan Nguyen using MAC (left), Lina Dahlbeck using MAC (right) **Styling:** Karl Willett **Models:** Alex Beer and Anthony Lowther. Skull by Butler & Wilson, head piece stylist's own

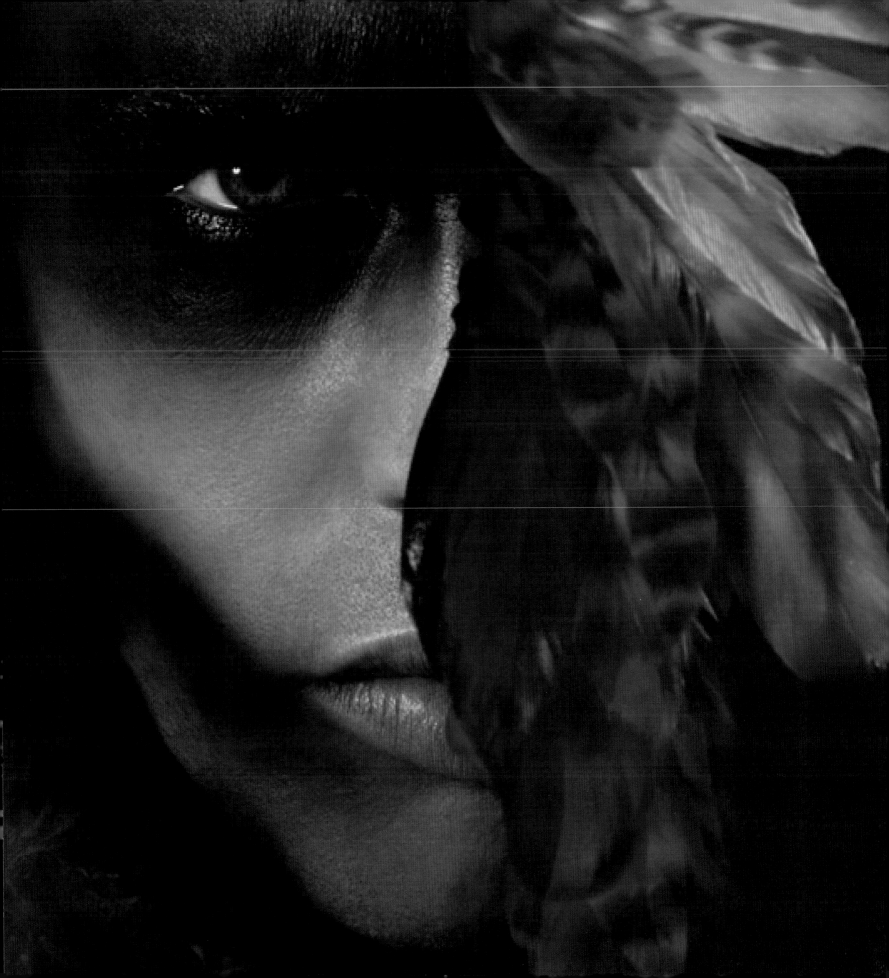

ICONIC ERAS

Prior to 1920, wearing makeup could be a dangerous proposition. It contained chemicals such as lead, sulphur and mercury. Beyond the health risks, it was not proper for nice girls to wear makeup. Those who did wore pale, muted colours and their supplies were hidden away from disapproving fathers and husbands. Women who feared the consequences of wearing makeup often vigorously pinched their cheeks and lips to give them colour. The prevailing attitude was that a lady had no reason to be in the sun and therefore should be pale. Some historians even suspect that the look became popular because of the prevalence of tuberculosis, which made its sufferers look very pallid.

The 1920s flapper, the 1940s brow, the 1950s Marilyn Monroe vamp and the 1960s Twiggy: all these, and other iconic makeup styles, are used over and over in film and fashion. Every year there seems to be another revival. Fashion designers take inspiration from the past, foreign cultures and street fashion and bring old trends to life with a new twist. The same goes for the makeup companies. New colours, products and techniques are brought back and re-introduced. We see brightly coloured lips all over the catwalks one season and Gothic black eyes the next.

The 1920s and 1930s were all about the dark and defined, with smoky eyes and bee-stung lips. In recent years, we have seen this look on numerous catwalk shows, like those created by Pat McGrath at Galliano for Dior. In the 1920s, eyebrows were kept natural and unplucked, while eyes were dark and smoky. The "smoky eye" is still one of the most popular makeup looks today. The incredibly beautiful actress Louise Brooks, called LuLu, was one of the fashion and beauty icons of the decade with her trademark Dutch bob and dramatic makeup, while Greta Garbo set the trend in the 1930s with plucked and drawn-in brows.

The 1940s, the swing era but more remembered for World War II, saw women join the workforce when their men were off at war. Looks were simplified; the red lipstick was a necessity. Lips were true red with the top lip overdrawn and rounded, heavy eyeliner was flicked at the outer corners and eyebrows were kept natural. A good example of the look of the time was the movie star Veronica Lake.

The glamorous Hollywood look of the 1950s is still current and trendy, with the pin-up, Marilyn Monroe look being adapted by the likes of Christina Aguilera, Scarlett Johansson and Dita von Teese, to name just a few. During this decade there was a transformation from the ponytailed, innocent teenage look to heavily-styled, beehive hair and defined eyes. Starlets wore red lipstick, eyeliner, blusher and lots of mascara; eyebrows were kept natural and grown out. Teenagers started wearing pink- and peach-coloured lipstick, as parents didn't approve of the heavily made-up looks.

The 1960s saw a complete change in makeup trends. Twiggy was discovered in 1966 and changed the world of fashion and beauty with her short, androgynous hair-do and Mod fashions created by such designers as Mary Quant. Twiggy wore light pastel lipstick and eyeshadow, false eyelashes, thick eyeliner drawn into her socket lines, and lots and lots of mascara. Mary Quant is just one of many designers who take credit for inventing the miniskirt and hot pants, but by the middle of the decade, she had brought out a new, trendy makeup line that offered multi-use products and palettes. The end of the 1960s was the beginning of the flower-power era and women's liberation, and makeup was minimal and natural. Hair was left long and unstyled and, not surprisingly, cosmetics companies struggled.

The 1970s saw a mix of glam rock, disco and punk music that soon spiced up the world of fashion and beauty. Clothes were fitted, trousers flared and unisex looks were introduced. Makeup was bold and garish and lots of colour and glitter was used. French and Italian *Vogue* showed

The 1920s Look

The look, as re-created right, was dark, mysterious and vamp, with heavy kohl-rimmed eyes and a cupid bow-mouth. Round shapes were created in the brow and eyes, with pink blush on the apple of the cheeks and rosebud dark lips. The brow shape starts straight, then rounds.

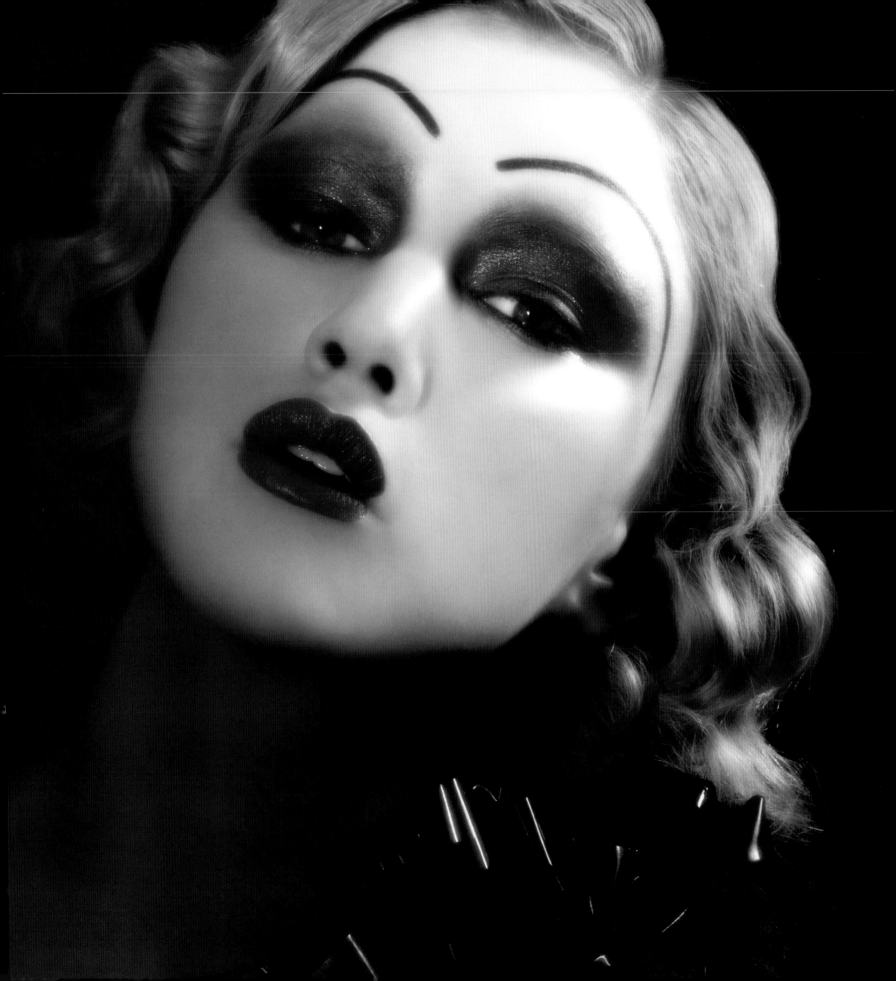

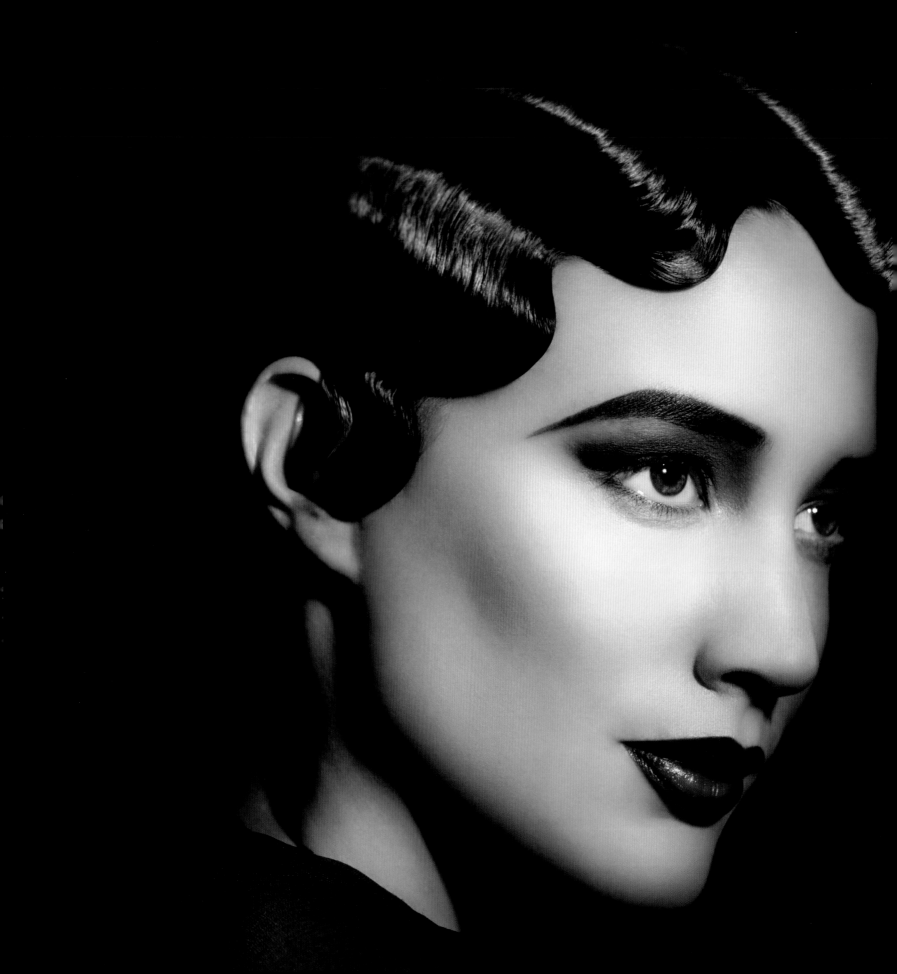

models wearing blood-red lipstick, black eye makeup and pencil-thin eyebrows. David Bowie and Roxy Music were the faces of glam rock. The makeup was correspondingly bold, colourful and above all, theatrical. Punk music and the anarchy movement dominated the end of the decade's social scene: safety pins became nose and ear jewellery and hair was harshly dyed, styled and sculpted into mohawks or spikes. Vivienne Westwood and her partner Malcolm McLaren created the iconic Sex Pistols look.

The 1980s saw an explosion of colour. Big and eccentric hairstyles and makeup looks were popularized by television, film and music stars. Shows such as *Dynasty*, *Miami Vice* and *Fame,* coupled with major artists like Michael Jackson and Madonna, were just a few of the influences. Duran Duran and Adam and the Ants were the faces of the New Romantic scene and experimented with androgynous looks.

Hair was worn big and frizzy by both sexes throughout the 1980s and lots of hair products were used, while makeup was colourful and bold. The fluoro colours of fashion were replicated in the makeup of the time, with women wearing brightly coloured mascaras and bold eyeshadows, blended up to the brow. Blushers were also applied in excess and blended to the hairline.

Throughout this chapter you will see a range of different retro makeup looks from the 1920s through to the current trends. You can imitate them if you like, or simply be inspired by the amazing way the past can inject energy into a look.

The 1930s Look

The look for this decade, see left, was elegant and sophisticated, with softer eyeshadow, a blended socket with heavy lashes and mascara. Blush is sculpted on the cheek. Fuller lips slope from the bow. The brow shape is rounded from start to finish.

1 Apply a tinted moisturizer or light-coverage foundation all over face. Touch up any imperfections or dark circles with a concealer. Apply concealer or eyeshadow primer on the eyelids as a base.

2 Using a soft black eyeliner, draw a thick line along the upper lash line. You can also use a black cream eyeshadow for this. Using your fingers or a synthetic brush, smudge the line up to the socket then apply a black eyeshadow on top to set. Using a soft brush, blend the colour toward the socket.

3 Apply a light grey or dusky brown in the sockets to help the black blend into the browbone area.

4 Leave the browbone as it is and set with a translucent powder, or apply a highlighter up to the eyebrow.

5 Curl the lashes. Apply plenty of black mascara.

6 Brush the eyebrows into place and define them using an eyebrow shadow or pencil. Set the shape using a clear brow fix.

7 The look is all about the dramatic eyes and lips, so keep the cheeks as natural as possible with just a touch of peach blusher on the outer corners of the apples of the cheeks. Blend it up toward the temples and follow with a pressed powder contouring shadow in natural in the hollows of the cheeks to create depth and shape.

8 Line the lips with a dark burgundy lipliner, then fill in lips with the same pencil. Blend with a clean lip brush before applying a matching matte lipstick on top. Alternatively, for a more modern twist, use gloss or a lipstick with a slight sheen instead of the matte lipstick.

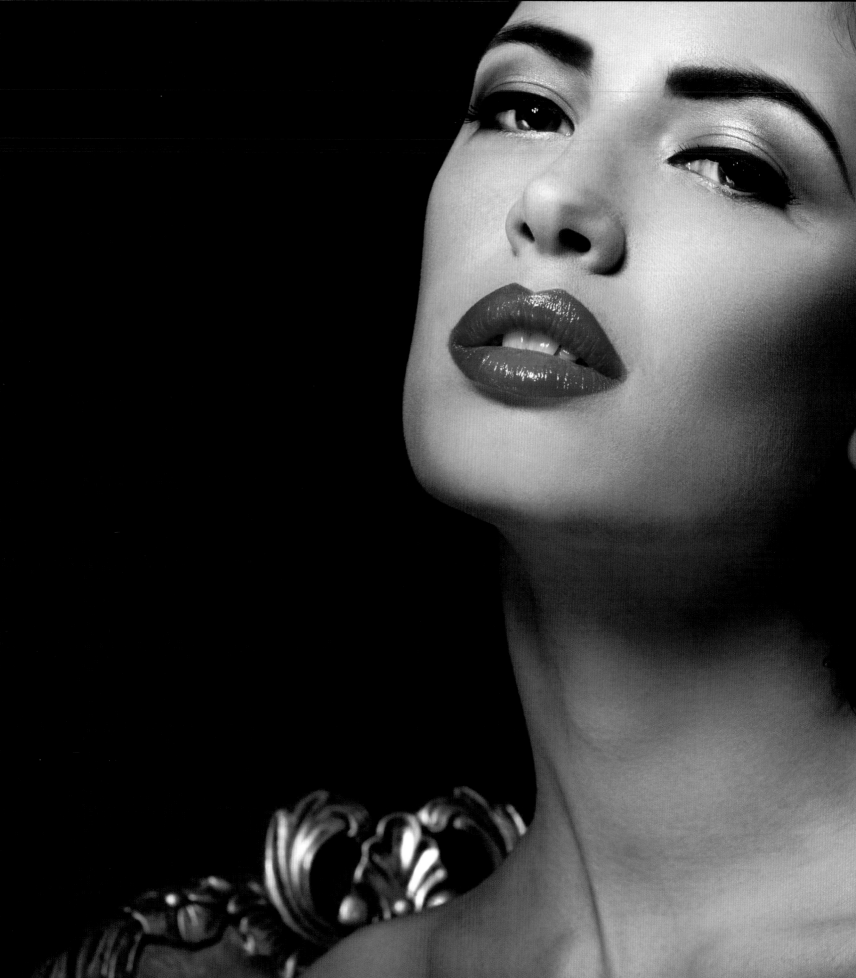

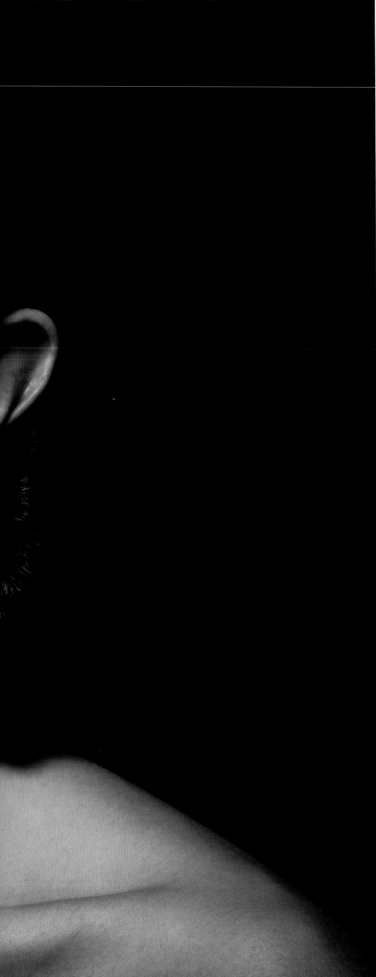

Photographer:
Catherine Harbour
Makeup: Rachel
Wood using Chanel
Hair: Marc Eastlake
using Bumble & Bumble
Model: Sabrina @ Next

The 1940s Look

Period makeup was minimal, classic and elegant.
To re-create the look, taupe socket eyeshadow
was used with liner smudged through the fine
lashes. Blush was sculpted on the cheek and red
lips were fuller and wider at the bow. The brows
were long and arched.

The 1950s Look

Glamorous, clean and fresh, the eyes were pastel – blue, pink and violet. Eyeliner was used in an Egyptian shape for a classic 1950s flick. In this decade false eyelashes were used, and lips were a lighter red, pink or orange. Blush in pinks and peaches were sculpted on the apples of the cheeks and the brow was strong and arched.

The look here was inspired by the original Barbie-doll look, mixed with *I Love Lucy's* Lucille Ball. Wide eyes were painted with a powder-blue shadow, white eyeliner was applied on the inside of the eye and black liquid liner – thicker in the middle of the eye – was applied across the lid. A touch of white loose shimmer eyeshadow on the middle of the lid created a touch of high glamour. False eyelashes were applied to the top eyelash.

A classic red pout was created with the bottom lip drawn on slightly smaller than the top lip, producing an innocent, Barbie-doll pout. The warm tone foundation was kept matte and heavy so the look has a B-movie, colourama effect.

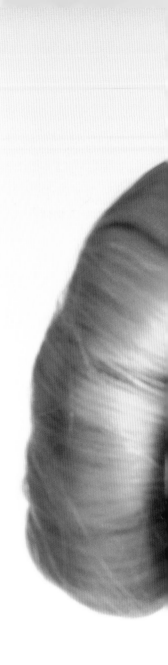

Photographer: Keith Clouston **Makeup:** Rachel Wood using Benefit **Hair:** Fabio Vivian **Model:** Invlid @ mandpmodels

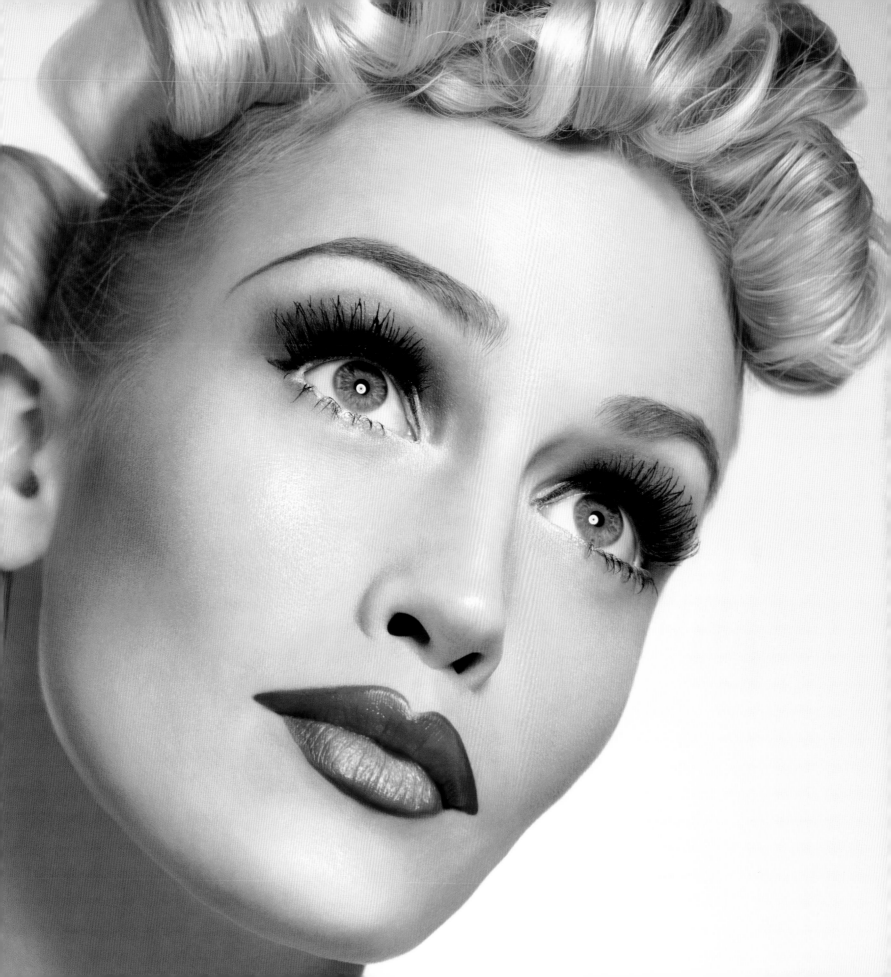

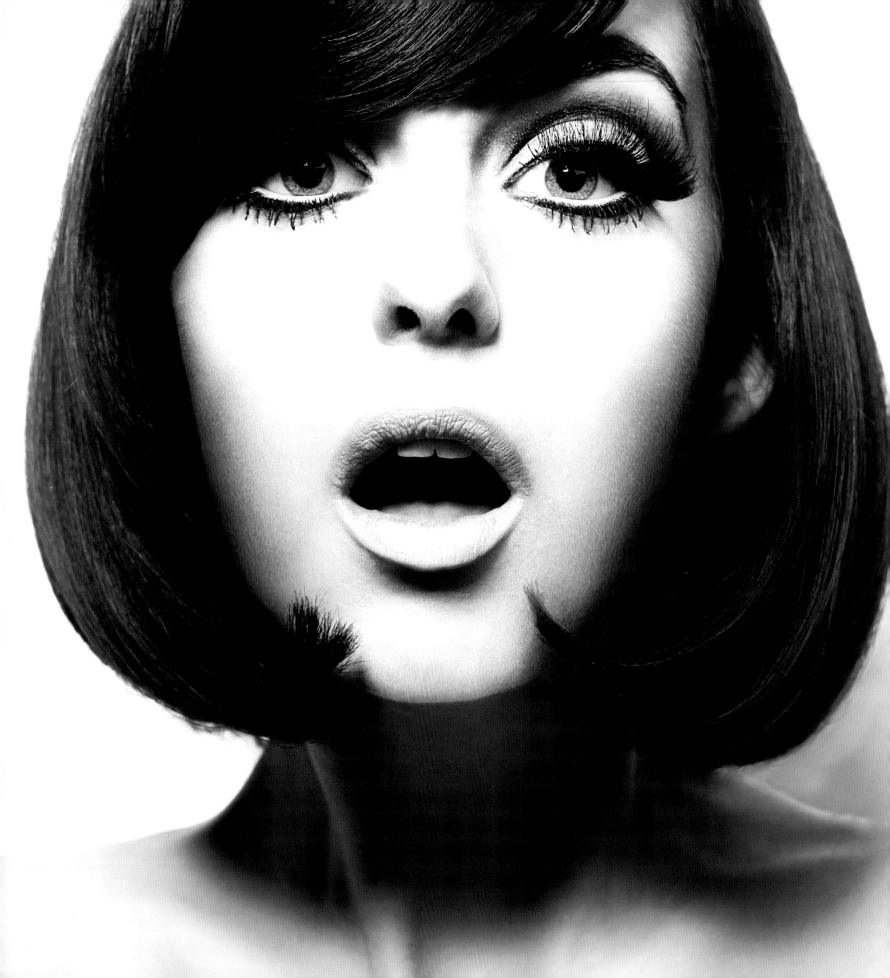

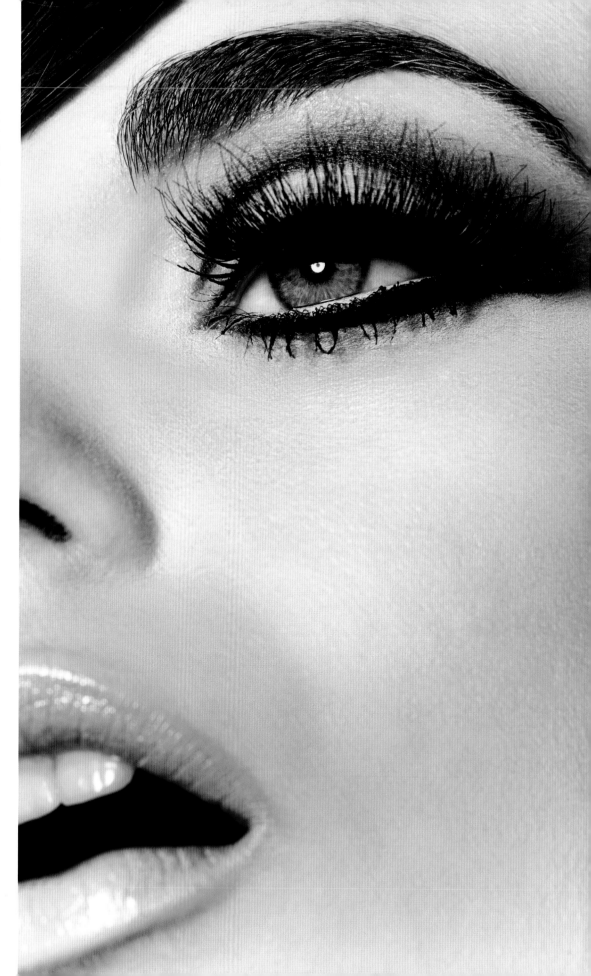

The 1960s Dollybird Look

The pale face "dollybird" look reigned supreme. Eyes were pale with strong liner applied top and bottom and charcoal upper lids, with heavy false lashes. Heavy highlighter and sculpted blush were used, and lips were in pale brown, soft pinks and peaches.

The look here was inspired by Andy Warhol, Twiggy and a touch of over-the-top Austin Powers. A combination of black wet/dry powder liner and matte white eyeshadow were used to create a graphic eye. Four layers black mascara were applied to the eyelashes, then a very thick pair of fluffy false eyelashes were added on top to finish the look.

Photographer:
Catherine Harbour
Makeup: Rachel
Wood using Benefit
Hair: Marc Eastlake
using Bumble & Bumble
Model: Viktoria @
Oxygen

Photographer: Lou
Denim **Makeup:**
Cristina Iravedra
using Kryolan
Model: Eline @
manadp models

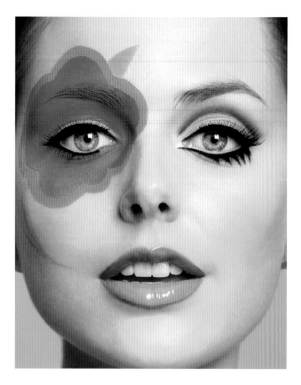

The 1960s Pop-Art Look

Based on the iconic image of the 1960s model Twiggy by Richard Avedon, this great style, seen above, can be adapted for a party look.

1 Apply a light foundation, such as MAC Face and Body, all over the face, making sure to cover any dark circles with a medium-to-heavy cream concealer. Blend foundation on the ears and into the neck and chest area.

2 Next, apply loose translucent powder to set the foundation and avoid shine later on.

3 Apply a light/pale grey matte eyeshadow all over eyelids, then add a dark grey/black matte eyeshadow over the eye crease to create a "banana" effect. Blend the dark colour well, but make sure that it is still well defined. Only use the dark colour on the right eye, as the left one will be painted.

4 Curl the eyelashes.

5 Using a thin, short eyeliner brush, apply black gel eyeliner on the right eye, contouring the eye and making sure the tear duct area is free of product. Flick the line upwards at the outside top corner. Along the bottom make a few spikes or flicks downward to create a false eyelash effect.

6 Apply eyeliner to the left eye, but do not add flicks along the bottom line.

7 Apply a white eye pencil all over the inner line of both eyes. This will make the eyes look dramatically bigger and will intensify the liner and the eye shape.

8 Add spiked false eyelashes on top of the natural ones, sticking them on with surgical eyelash glue. If the eyelashes are too big, cut them to size before adding the glue.

9 Apply black mascara with a zigzag motion to blend both real and false lashes.

10 Apply a peach blusher on the cheekbones with a circular motion.

11 Line the lips with a peach/orange lipliner, following the natural contour of the lips. Using a lip brush, fill in with peach lip gloss.

12 To draw the flower, use acrylic brushes (available from art shops) and Kryolan Aquacolors in blue, orange and pale green. Mix the dry paint with water until you get a creamy consistency.

13 First paint the blue inner colour, creating the main flower shape (be really careful around the eye). Contour the shape with orange colour, using a thinner brush. Draw on the green leaf with a fine brush.

The 1960s Op-Art Look

Inspired by a Paco Rabanne earring created in the late 1960s, this period look, see right, is made contemporary with the addition of a graphic design. On the face peach powder blush is used with beige sculpting powder and a creamy neutral coral beige lipstick is used on the lips. Gel/cream liners in pure white and black are used with matte white and black eyeshadow to create the eye design.

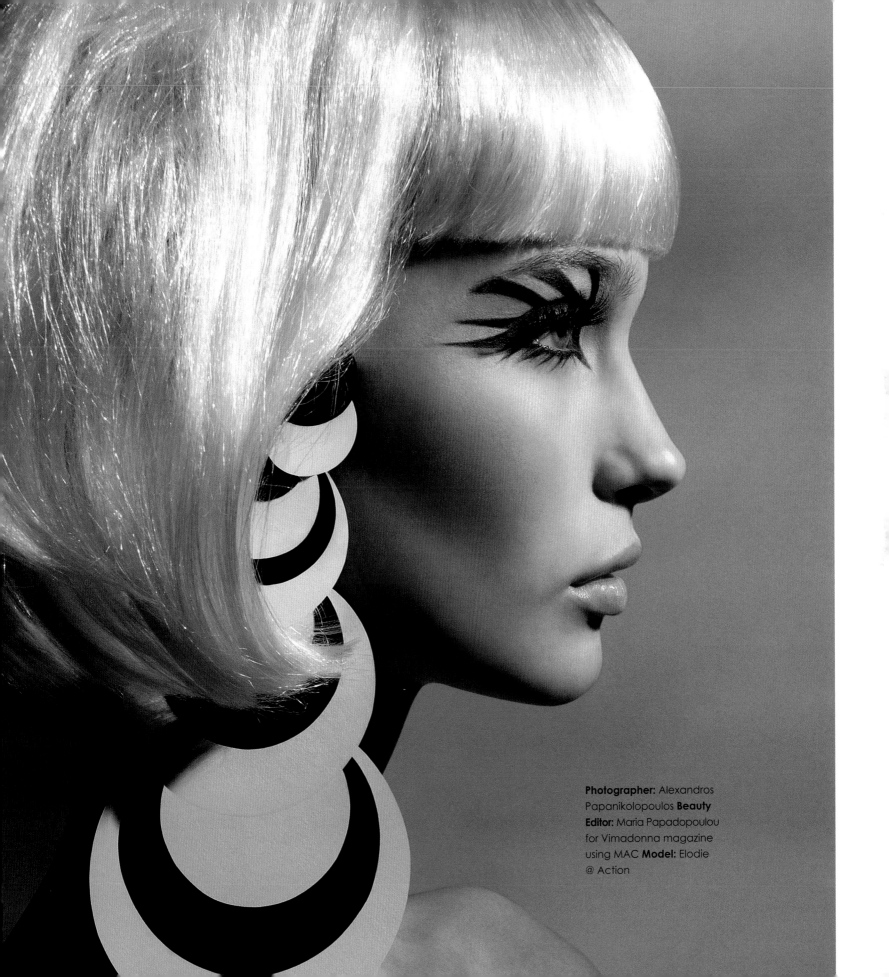

Photographer: Alexandros Papanikolopoulos **Beauty Editor:** Maria Papadopoulou for Vimadonna magazine using MAC **Model:** Elodie @ Action

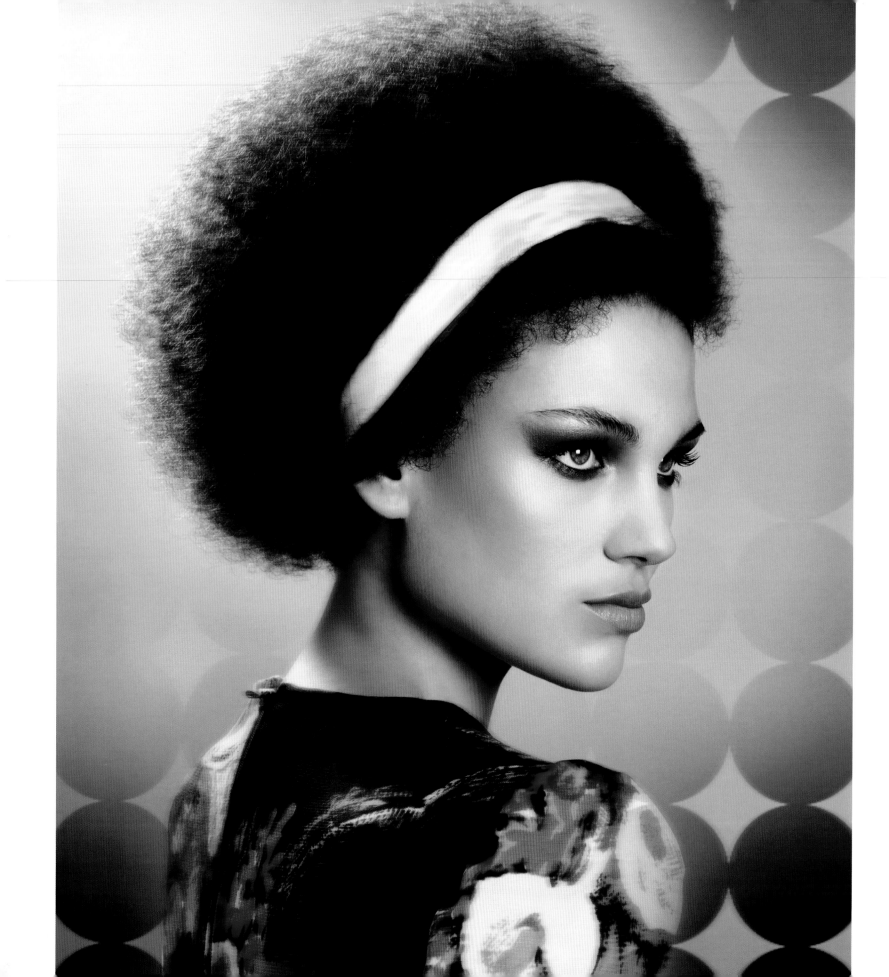

The 1970s Look

Colourful, natural face painting created a tanned look and highlighting and shading were used to sculpt the look, as seen left. Eyes were colourful, with pencils used for definition, and in iridescent shadow textures. Lips were very glossy and brows were thin with a slight arch.

1 Apply a tinted moisturizer or light-coverage foundation all over face, making sure to touch up any imperfections or dark circles with a concealer. Use a concealer or eyeshadow primer on the eyelids.

2 Next add a light green eyeshadow to the lids and, using a soft blending brush, blend toward the socket.

3 Apply a tan/brown eyeshadow to the sockets of the eye and blend up toward the middle of the browbone area. Highlight the eyes using a shimmery gold shadow on the browbone under the brows.

4 Give the eyes, and the whole look, more depth and drama by applying black eyeliner along the upper and lower lash lines Blend with a small brush and set with dark green eyeshadow.

5 Curl the lashes and apply black mascara.

6 Brush the eyebrows in place and define them using an eyebrow shadow or pencil, then set the shape using a clear brow fix.

7 Define the cheekbones by applying bronzer and blending up toward the temples. Add a pressed powder contouring shadow in a natural tone to the hollows of the cheeks to create depth and shape.

8 Line the lips with a barely-there beige lipliner. Blend the edges using your fingers or a lip brush and apply a clear lip gloss on top.

9 Finish with a dusting of translucent powder.

Photographer: Lou Denim
Makeup: Lina Dahlbeck
using Kryolan **Model:**
Emma Cantaloup @ Union

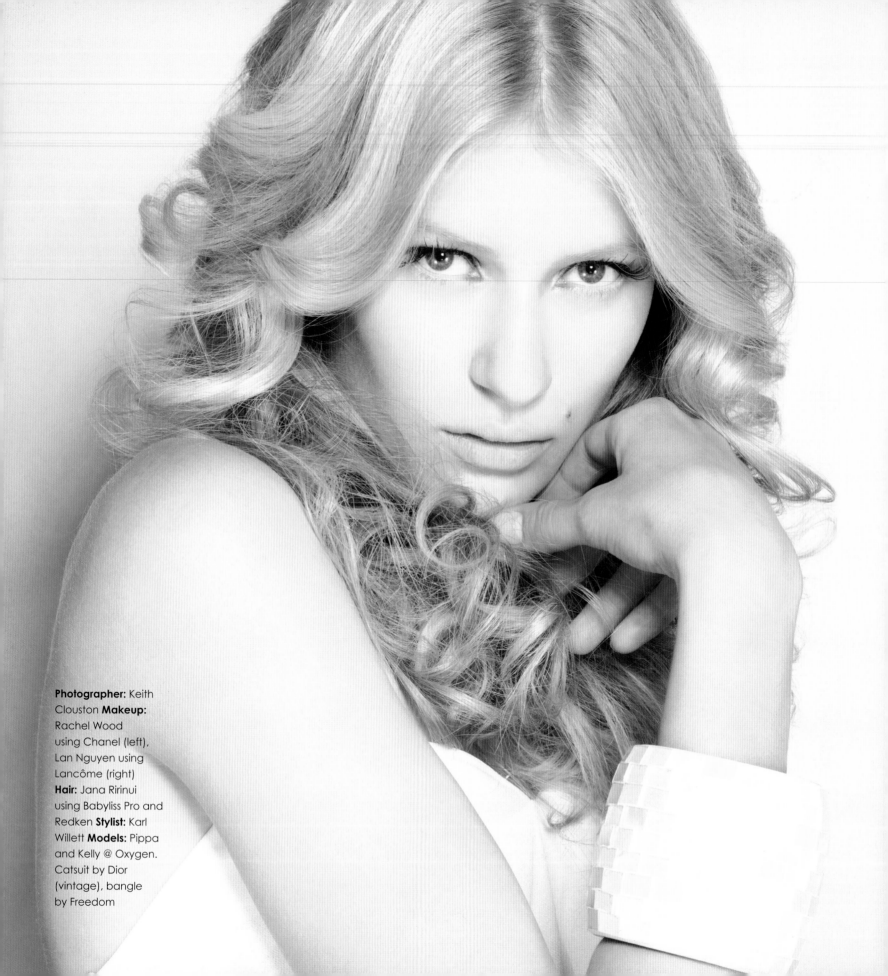

Photographer: Keith Clouston **Makeup:** Rachel Wood using Chanel (left), Lan Nguyen using Lancôme (right) **Hair:** Jana Ririnui using Babyliss Pro and Redken **Stylist:** Karl Willett **Models:** Pippa and Kelly @ Oxygen. Catsuit by Dior (vintage), bangle by Freedom

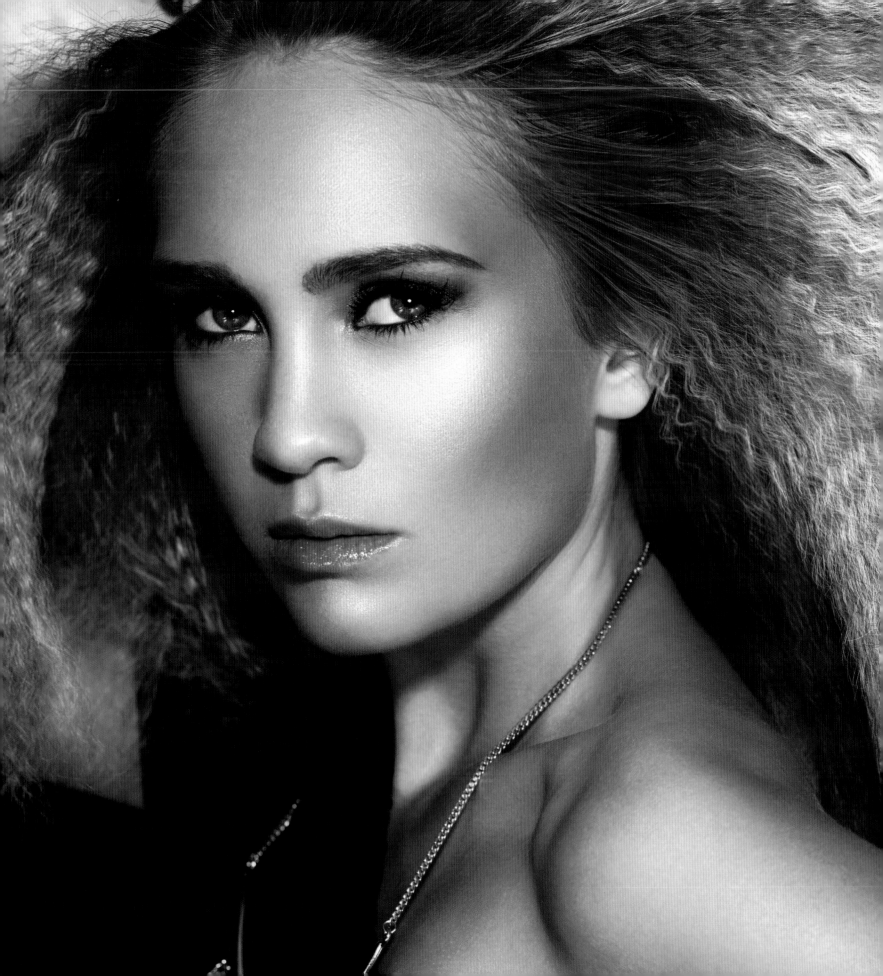

Photographer: Keith Clouston **Makeup and Hair:** Lan Nguyen using MAC and L'Oréal Professional **Stylist:** Karl Willett **Model:** Pippa @ Oxygen. Dress by Lucy Wrightwick, vintage gloves by Gucci

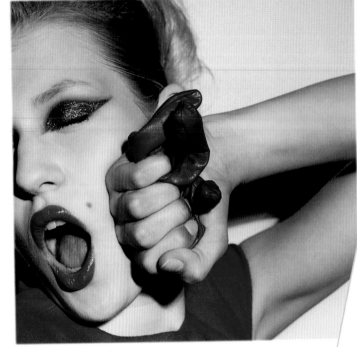

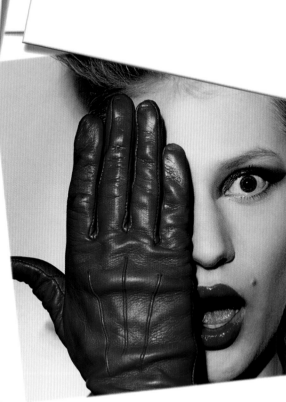

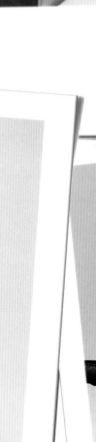

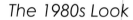

The 1980s Look

Matte, strong, serious and glamorous, 1980s makeup uses definition on eyes with a deep blended socket and liner top and bottom. Power red or shocking pink lipstick with natural heavy brows complete the look.

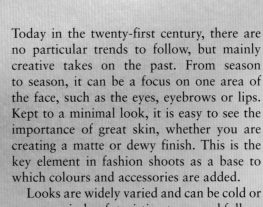

MODERN MILLENNIUM

Today in the twenty-first century, there are no particular trends to follow, but mainly creative takes on the past. From season to season, it can be a focus on one area of the face, such as the eyes, eyebrows or lips. Kept to a minimal look, it is easy to see the importance of great skin, whether you are creating a matte or dewy finish. This is the key element in fashion shoots as a base to which colours and accessories are added.

Looks are widely varied and can be cold or warm, period or futuristic, strong and full-on or soft and natural, finished or unfinished. It is the way in which makeup is applied and played with by the artist that defines what the look will be. It is importance is to achieve the right balance between being artistic and developing a commercial look that is beautiful, wearable and successful.

As new products come on the market, makeup artists must keep up to date with trends and develop an understanding of the new formulas. This ensures that the look you create is on trend. You can also be inspired to create interesting and new looks by mixing the colours you already have and using them differently on the face. For example, a bright-coloured cheek cream base, such as Shock Pink blush by MAC, could also be used on the lips and eyes to create a modern feel.

Photographer:
Catherine Harbour
Makeup: Lan Nguyen
using MAC **Model:** Ilize
Bajane @ Next

The Millennium Look

Today's looks are eclectic, varied and a combination of all the eras mixed into one. Metallic cream eyeshadows or greasepaints, glitters and strong colours give impact and foundation approaches, whether dewy or matte, can vary. Nowadays looks can be dictated by a designer, stylist, artist, magazine editor, art director or even a PR agent, as well as celebrities and the music industry.

1 Using a foundation brush, apply full-coverage foundation all over for a clean, flawless base.

2 With an eyeliner brush apply black gel liner on the entire eyelid up to the socket. Soften the edges and set with black shadow. Blend well.

3 Now line the inner eye rims with a white pencil. Add white gel liner, such as MAC Pure White, on the lower lash line and under the lash line from the inner corner to the outer corner to achieve a thick white line.

4 Draw black gel liner under the white liner and soften the edges.

5 Attach false lashes on upper lash only, sticking them on with eyelash glue.

6 Neaten eyebrows and fill in with an eyebrow pencil or shadow if necessary.

7 Softly contour under the cheekbones with a natural blush colour.

8 Apply a matte red lipstick to the lips and add a slick of clear gloss over the top.

Photographer: Lou Denim **Makeup:** Elesbeth Tan using MAC **Model:** Lucy Jacques @ Nevs

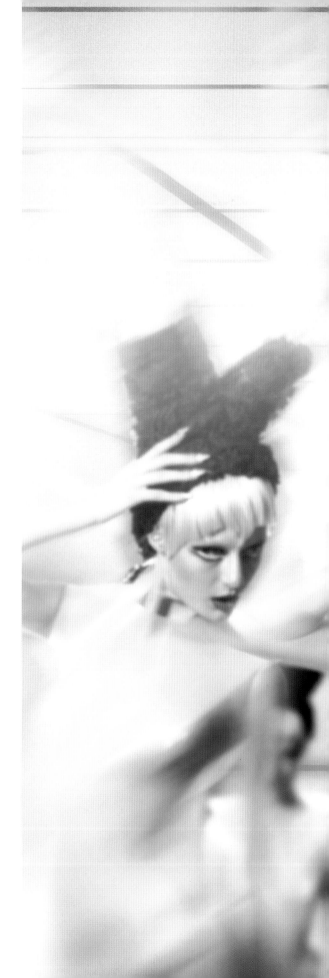

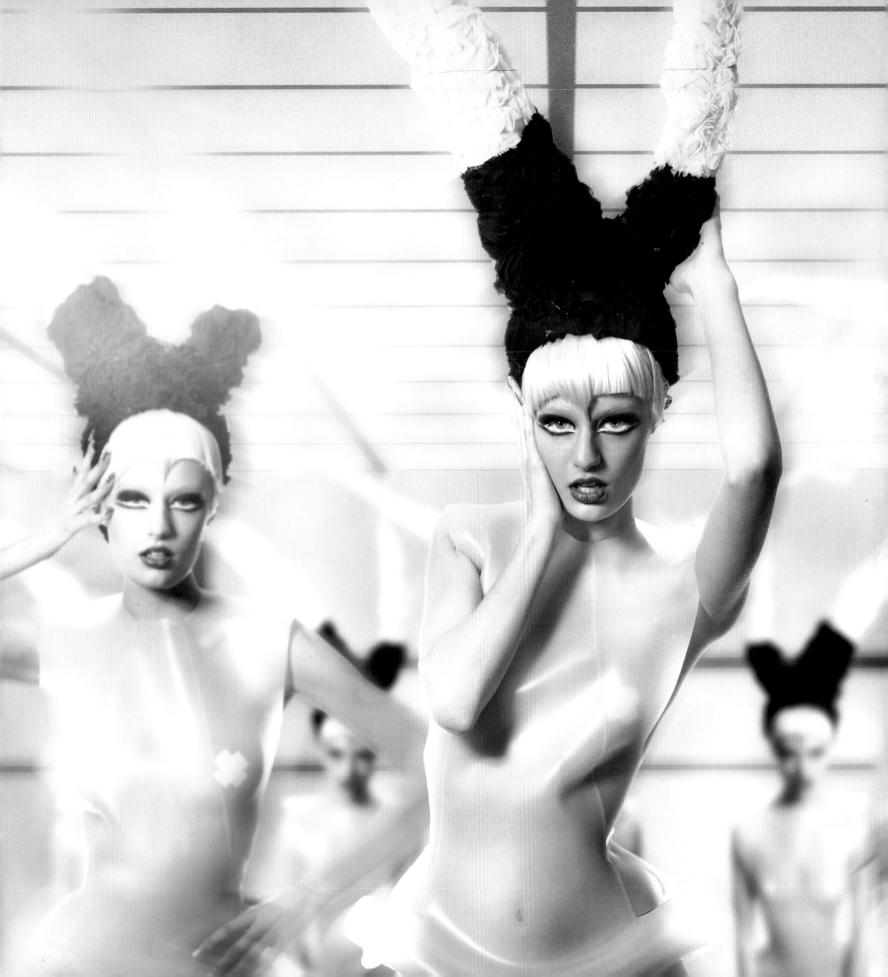

RED CARPET

When asked to do "red carpet" and celebrity makeup, there are many factors to take into consideration as the makeup is often dictated by the celebrity's personal preference or the image that they wish to project. It is essential to research your celebrity, or client, to see if they maintain a constant image or prefer to change their look regularly. Look at the makeup they use and see where you can improve their overall look and style.

Find out what event they will be attending, and, if possible, what they are wearing. Speak with the hairdresser and stylist to see what their ideas are and meet the client before the event to discuss what they want.

Be armed with tearsheets and printouts of your client and have a range of examples of what you will do so you can show the visuals and ensure you are using the same terminology. You may be called to the client's house, a hotel or a salon to do the makeup. Either way, it is a good idea to do a mini-facial before starting the makeup process. It also helps to wait about 10 minutes for the creams to be fully absorbed. This is an ideal time for the hairdresser to start working on the hair.

You should be able to complete your makeup within 30 minutes to an hour. The makeup is nearly always glamorous and you will often be asked to recreate the classic Hollywood look, so know your periods and what looks are popular with other celebrities. Be aware of current trends and be prepared to work at the same time as the hairdresser – celebrities are often late or working to a tight schedule. Check your work with your own camera. The makeup should be done to last the entire event, as you will not be on hand to do touch-ups later on.

Carry empty pots with you so you can give samples of the makeup you have used to the client, in case they want to touch-up themselves later. When you are working with a celebrity over a period of time, or if you are asked, be ready to advise them on which products they should have in their personal makeup bag. Companies will often give you free products for celebrities they want to be associated with.

Treat this type of makeup the same as you would photography work, as the paparazzi will be taking pictures at the event.

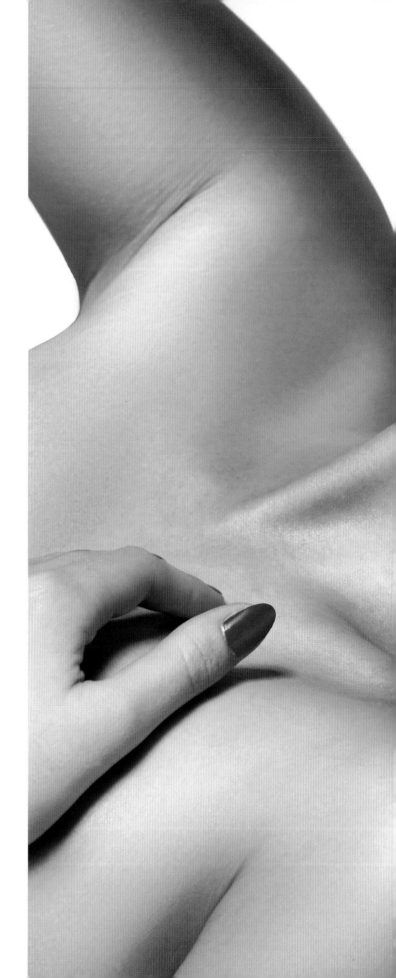

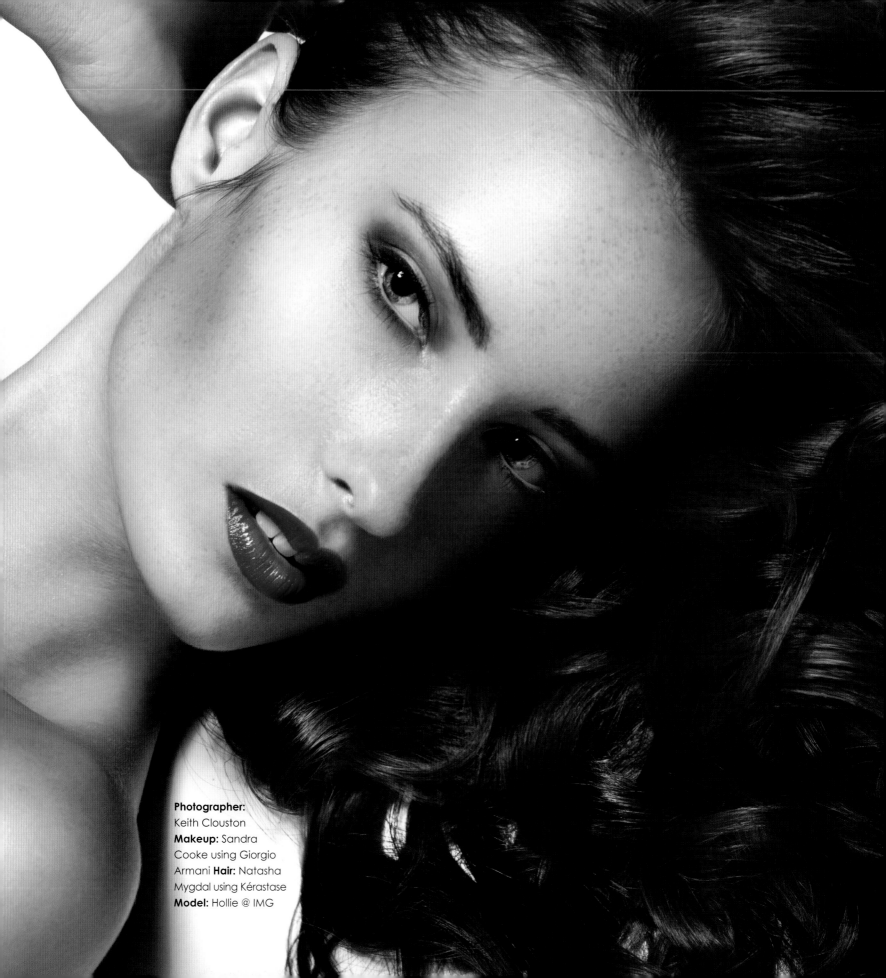

Photographer:
Keith Clouston
Makeup: Sandra
Cooke using Giorgio
Armani **Hair:** Natasha
Mygdal using Kérastase
Model: Hollie @ IMG

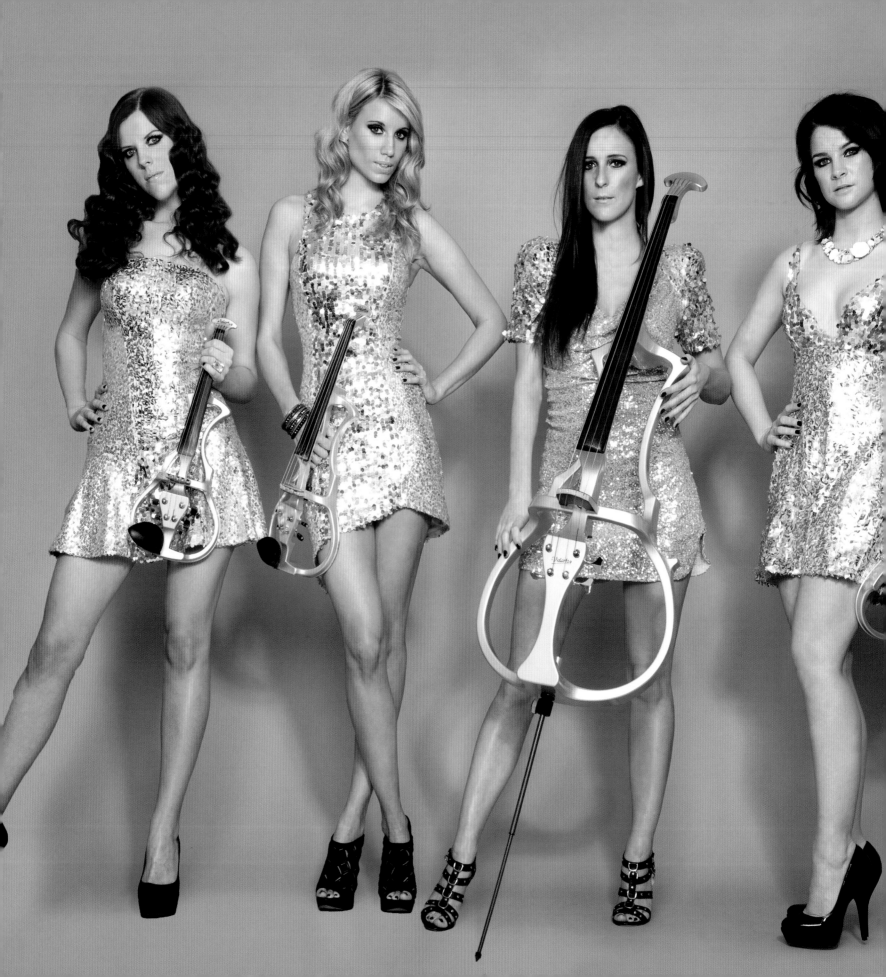

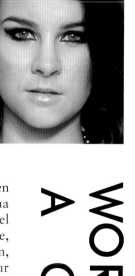

Celebrities always look immaculate and ooze "wow" factor, but it takes a little polishing here and there to make that possible. With cameras constantly flashing, the makeup needs to last all day and look good in strong light. As well as the red carpet, a celebrity might also hire a makeup artist for music videos, films, television and public appearances, so your personal relationship with them is very important – understanding their needs should be part of your work.

eScala Musical Group

Comprising, from left to right opposite, Chantal Leverton, viola player, cellist Tasya Hodges and violinists Izzy Johnston and Victoria Lyon, eScala are an electric string quartet who caused a sensation in the final of *Britain's Got Talent* in 2008. They performed in front of 14 million viewers on the show and were signed by Simon Cowell. Their debut album, produced by Trevor Horn, is available at www.escalamusic.com.

1 Working with a group requires a different approach to that of working with a single celebrity. First define their style as a group and then decide on a look that will enhance all their individual natural assets. Experiment with different hairstyles and makeup colours and play with numerous eye and lip shades.

2 For this shoot, the skin was prepped with Alpha-H Liquid Gold to tighten and moisture the skin. After this a silicone matte primer was applied to ensure that the skin tone was even and to help the makeup to last longer.

3 MAC Face and Body Foundation was mixed with a bit of full-coverage foundation with MAC Strobe Cream added to give a dewy look.

4 Never underestimate the value of eyes when achieving a star-studded look. To add drama a smoky eye was created using black gel liner, in this case MAC Blacktrack Fluidline, mixed with MAC's Bat Black Colour Cream, a blackened burgundy. A splash of colour eyeshadow, here MAC Blue Calm, was added on the edges to modernize the look.

5 For extra definition false eyelashes were applied and the line drawn over with black liquid liner.

6 To balance the eyes, you need to add lip colour, but be careful that the eyes and lips do not compete with each other. Here a nude colour, MAC Snob, was used with a touch of gloss on the centre of the lips to add sparkle.

WORKING WITH A GROUP

Photographer:
Catherine Harbour
Makeup: Lan Nguyen
using MAC Pro **Makeup**
Assistants: Elesbeth
Tan and Sharka P **Hair:**
Tim Furssedonn @ Toni
& Guy using Label M
Stylist: Rebekah Roy
Location: Inc Space

WORKING WITH AN ACTRESS

Tamsin Egerton

This shot is from an editorial shoot for *Urban Life* magazine, featuring actress and model Tamsin Egerton, best known for her role as Chelsea Parker in the *St Trinians* films (2007 and 2009). The magazine wanted to show her as a sophisticated woman and they had very clear, strong views on how to get this across. The team met before the shoot to discuss the ideas and how they would work together; each member had creative input to finalize a storyboard. The looks for the day, and the order to shoot them in, were talked through.

Photographer: Dez Mighty **Stylist:** Zed-Eye **Makeup:** Jo Sugar using Dermalogica and MAC **Hair:** Zach Jardin @ Neville

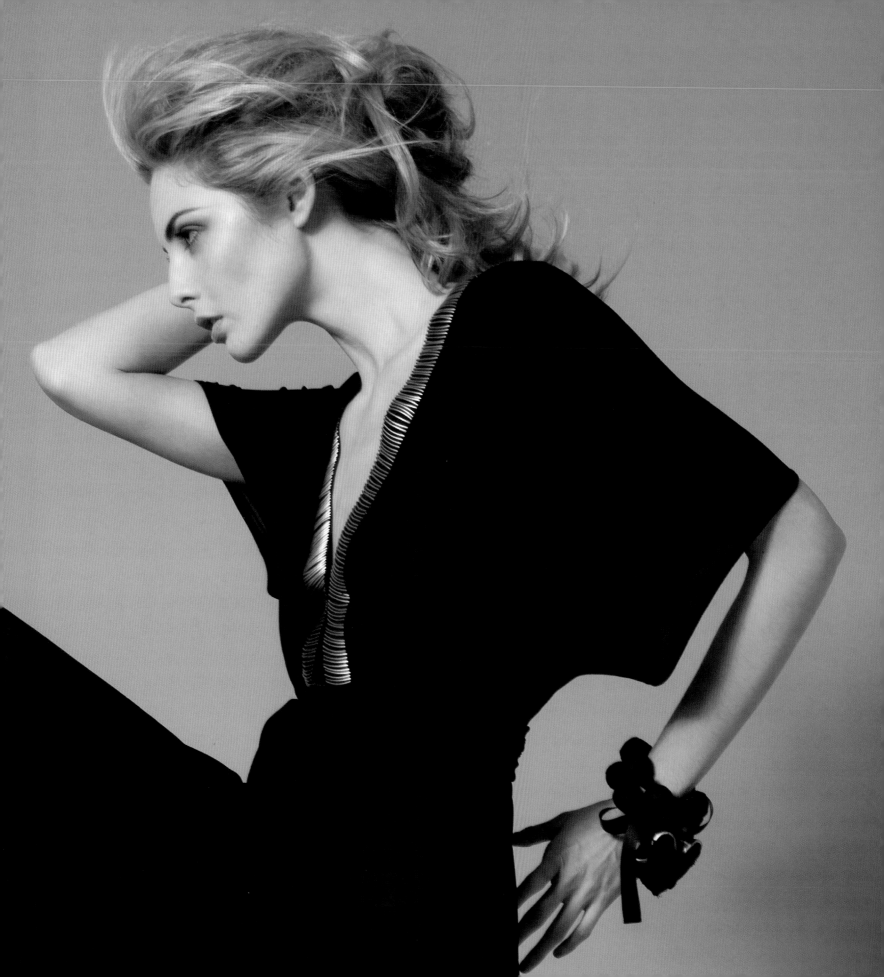

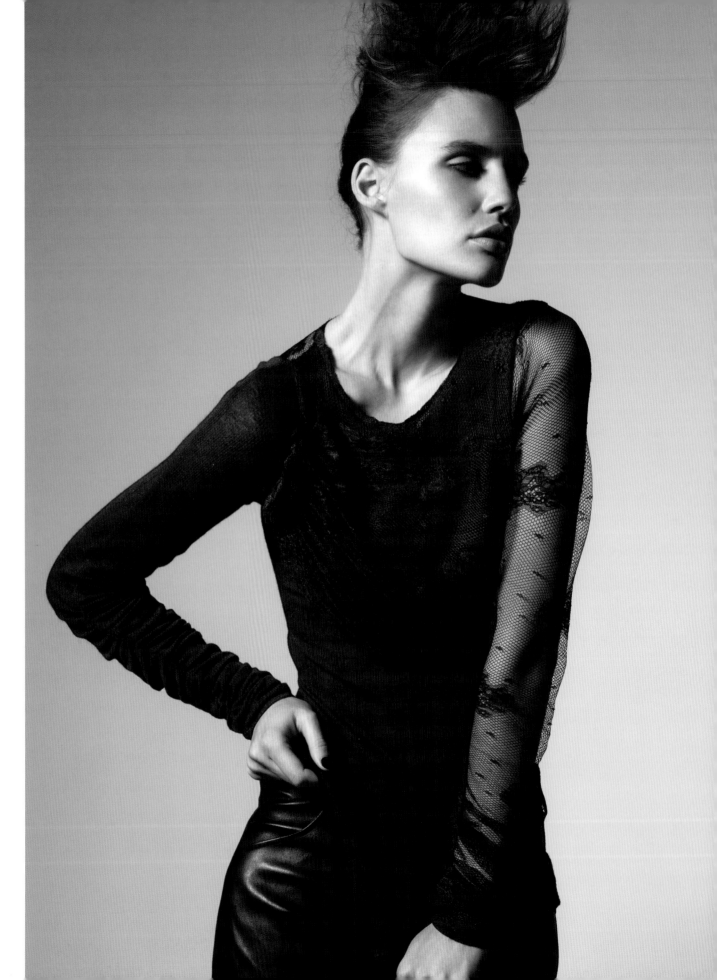

EDITORIAL

Photographer: Mo
Saito **Makeup:** Sandra
Cooke using Becca
Hair: Zoe Irwin @ Frank
Stylist: David Hawkins
@ Frank **Model:** Han-
nah @ Next

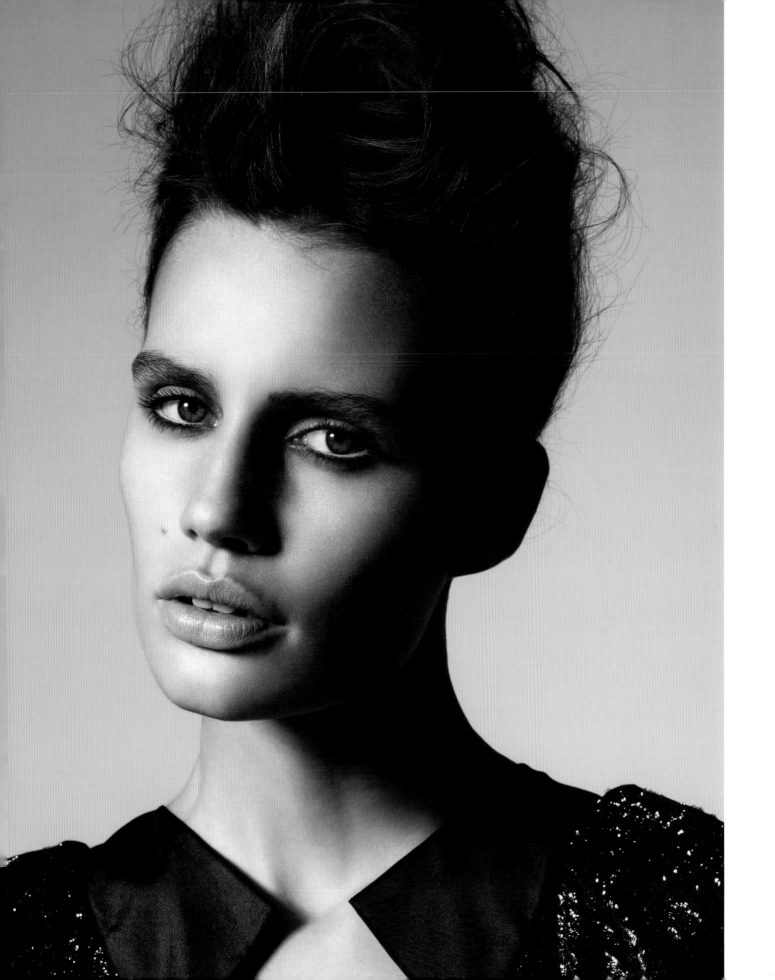

LIGHTING & MAKEUP

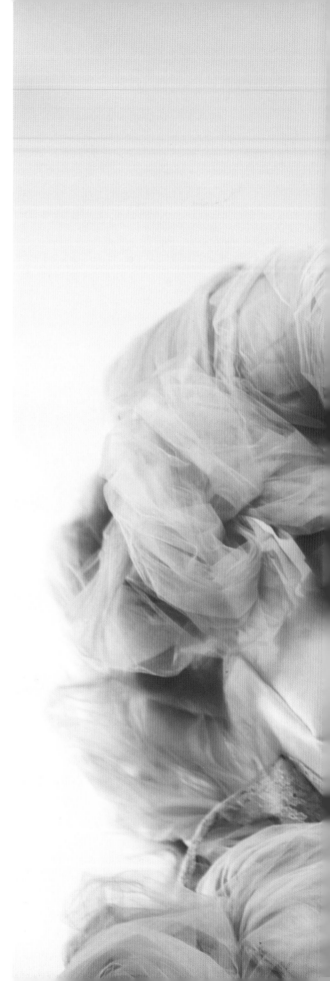

"There are so many elements that need to come together to produce a high-standard fashion editorial. Lots of planning and art direction, a good makeup artist, a stylist with the right clothing and accessories and the right models that are able to take direction and move well.

Some of the best editorial models are successful because they have a face like a blank canvas that can be moulded easily into any look. Lighting needs to be well thought-out, executed and tested on the model to make sure it complements her bone structure and shape.

Makeup is an integral part of the shoot, as it brings to life the concept and creates the look and feel of the model. Photographers will use the way the light bounces off the makeup to create a polished and beautiful result. A talented makeup artist will also know how to create perfect skin and reduce the amount of retouching needed later, thus creating a better-quality image. Editorial makeup often calls for a little more creativity and is a vehicle for pushing boundaries, new looks and techniques."

Camille Sanson, Photographer

"I am inspired by really strong makeup and one of the most important components of a fashion156. com shoot is to work with hugely creative makeup artists. Someone who really looks at the model's face and the clothing and then decides if their ideas are actually going to work. Sometimes initial ideas need to be scrapped and an equally strong idea needs to be conceptualized and produced within minutes. So many artists I meet want to play it safe. For me, eyes, lips and cheeks can all be strong on some (many!) occasions. Preconceived ideas and rules sometimes need to be broken!"

Guy Hipwell, Editor and Creative Director fashion156.com

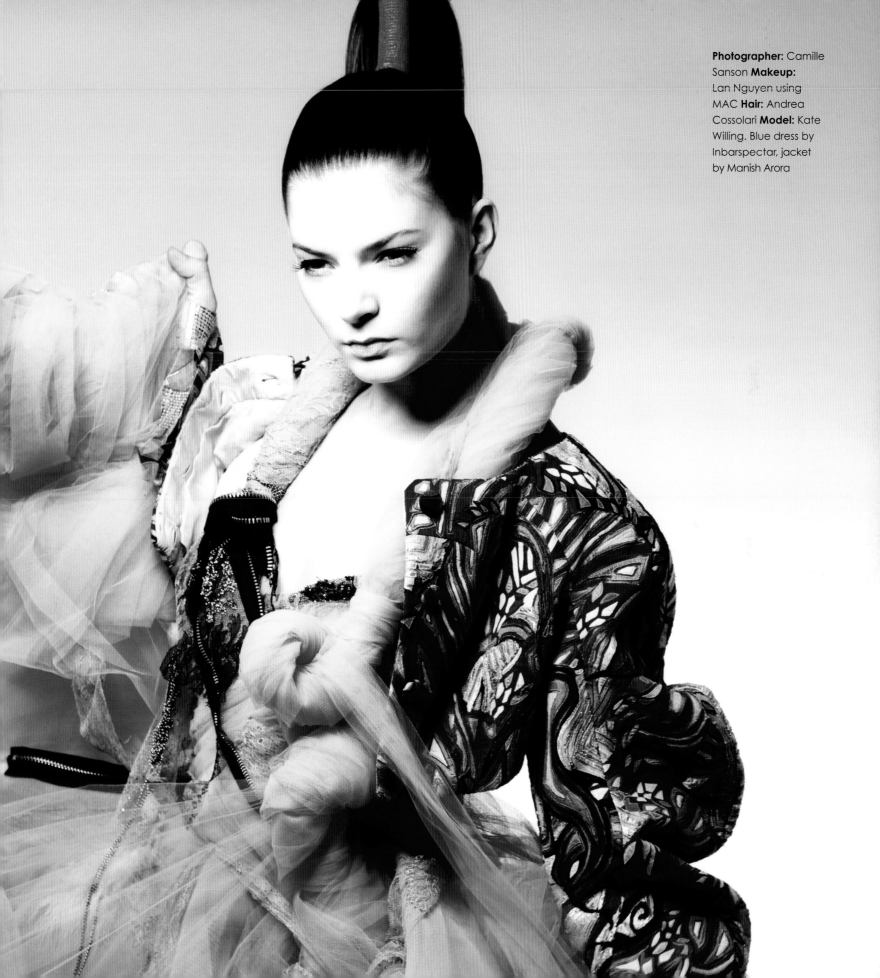

Photographer: Camille Sanson **Makeup:** Lan Nguyen using MAC **Hair:** Andrea Cossolari **Model:** Kate Willing. Blue dress by Inbarspectar, jacket by Manish Arora

STYLISTS & MAKEUP ARTISTS

"Let's just assume the makeup artist can do the basics – beautiful skin. And they are really creative. Then, the other qualities I think a makeup artist has to have is to be well organized, have a team they can trust, and they need to know about trends. Not just makeup trends, but also fashion and colour trends. A makeup artist, like the stylist, needs to be able to look at a selection of clothes and offer a variety of makeup looks. Often a junior makeup artist will ask 'What do you want?' I like a makeup artist who can offer suggestions and is not just an order taker. I'll make a mood board to give the team a vision and direction, but often the makeup artist will make one too. A beauty story can start with the vision of the makeup artist and they'll present a mood board. From there I can suggest the jewellery, accessories, etc.

I like to work with the same team because I can trust them. My work can be quite varied, from commercial to catwalk, so I need a makeup artist who is strong on many levels. He or she also needs to be personable. Once you know someone who can do the job it becomes all about personality – do you get along with them, are they the right fit? There are so many good makeup artists, so it can come down to having a similar vision – do they contribute to the team, are they responsible and fun to work with?"

Rebekah Roy, Fashion Stylist

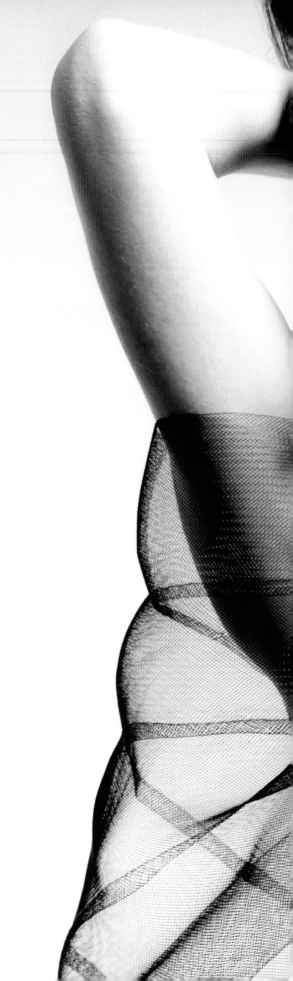

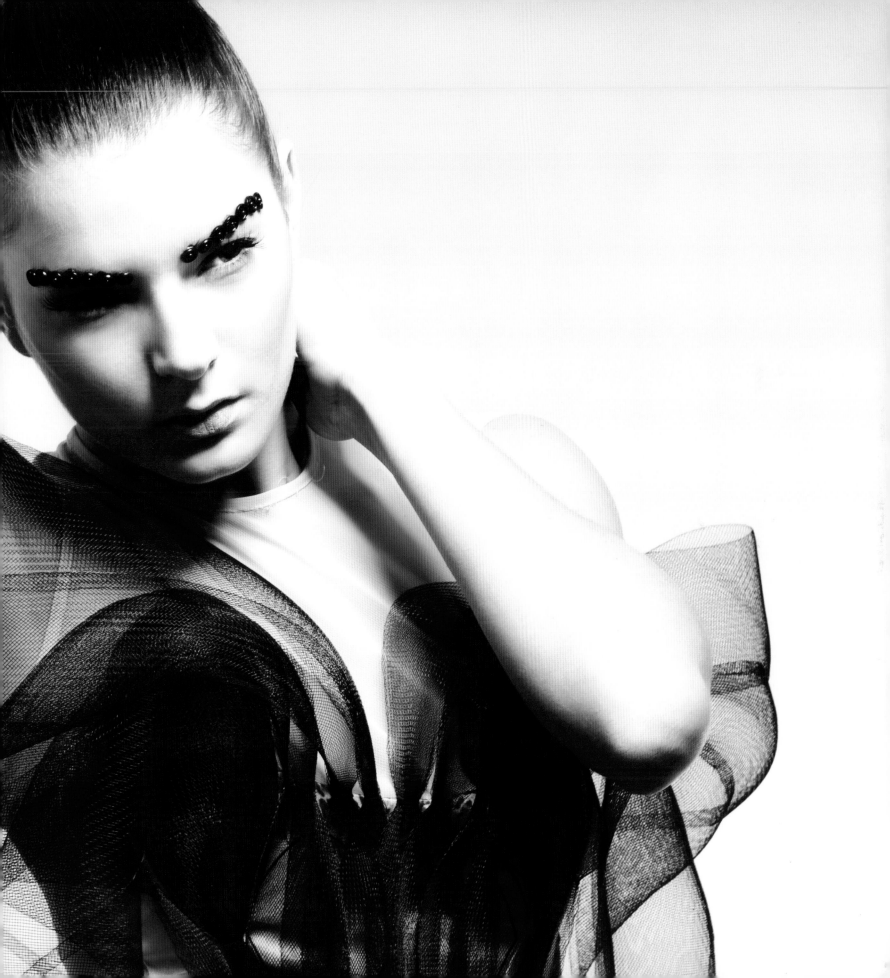

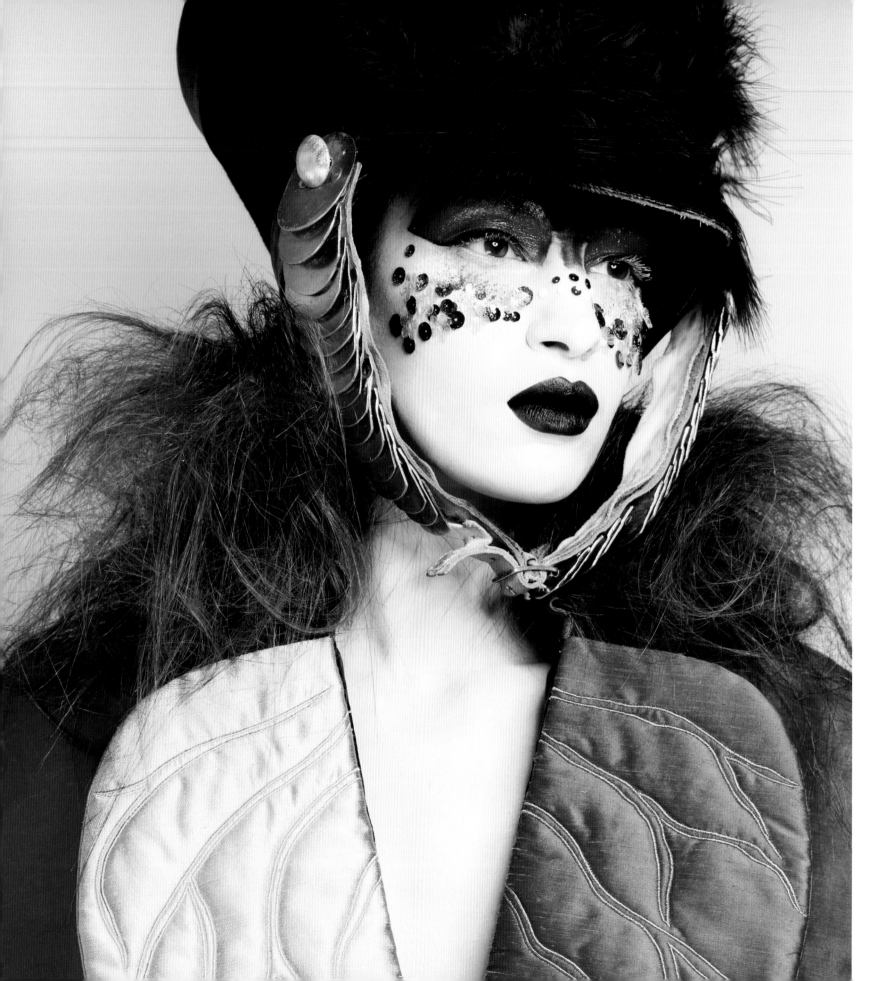

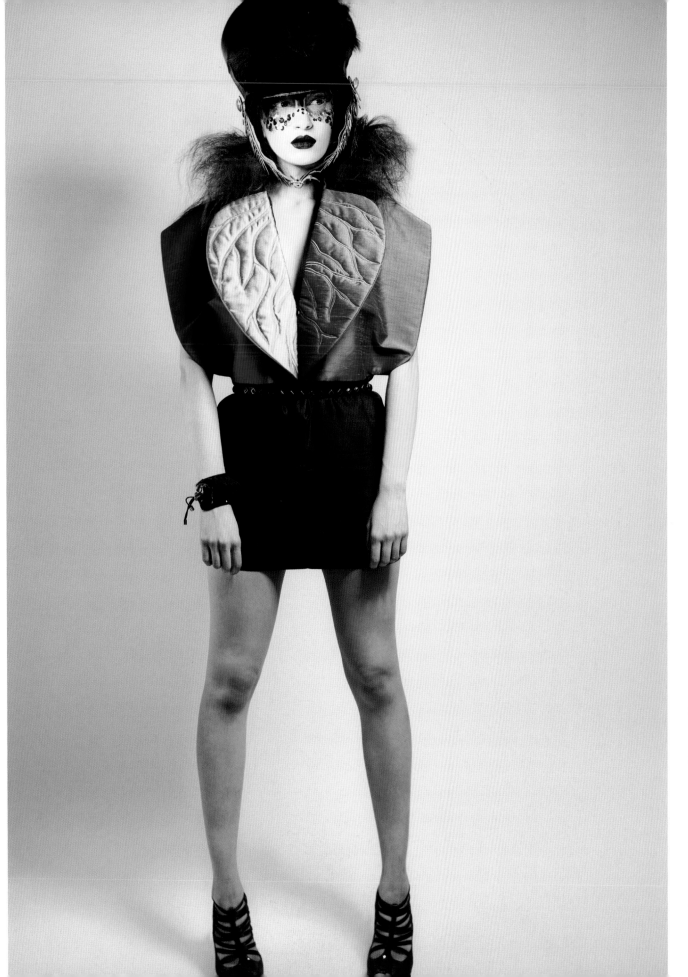

Photographer: Camille Sanson **Makeup:** Lan Nguyen using MAC **Hair:** Andrea Cassolari **Stylist:** Nasrin Jean-Baptiste **Model:** Elena @ Oxygen. Dress by Bernard Chandran, bracelet by J.W. Anderson, shoes by Modernist, all headwear customized by the stylist from a selection at Angels

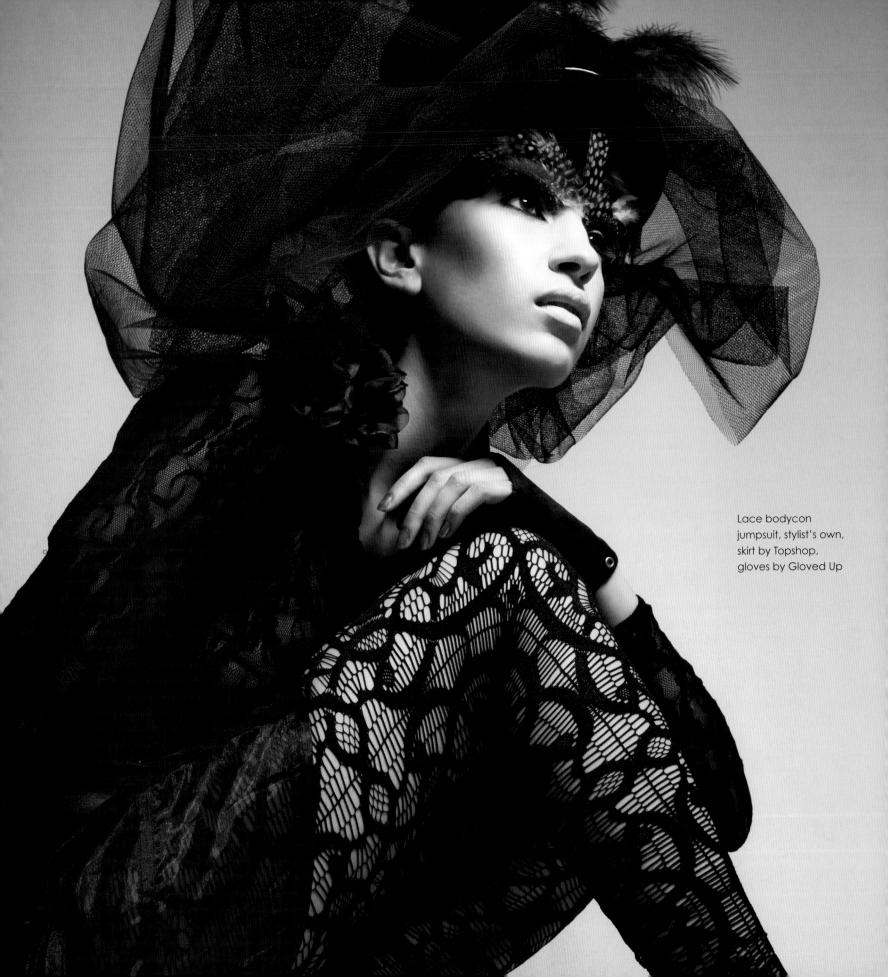

Lace bodycon
jumpsuit, stylist's own,
skirt by Topshop,
gloves by Gloved Up

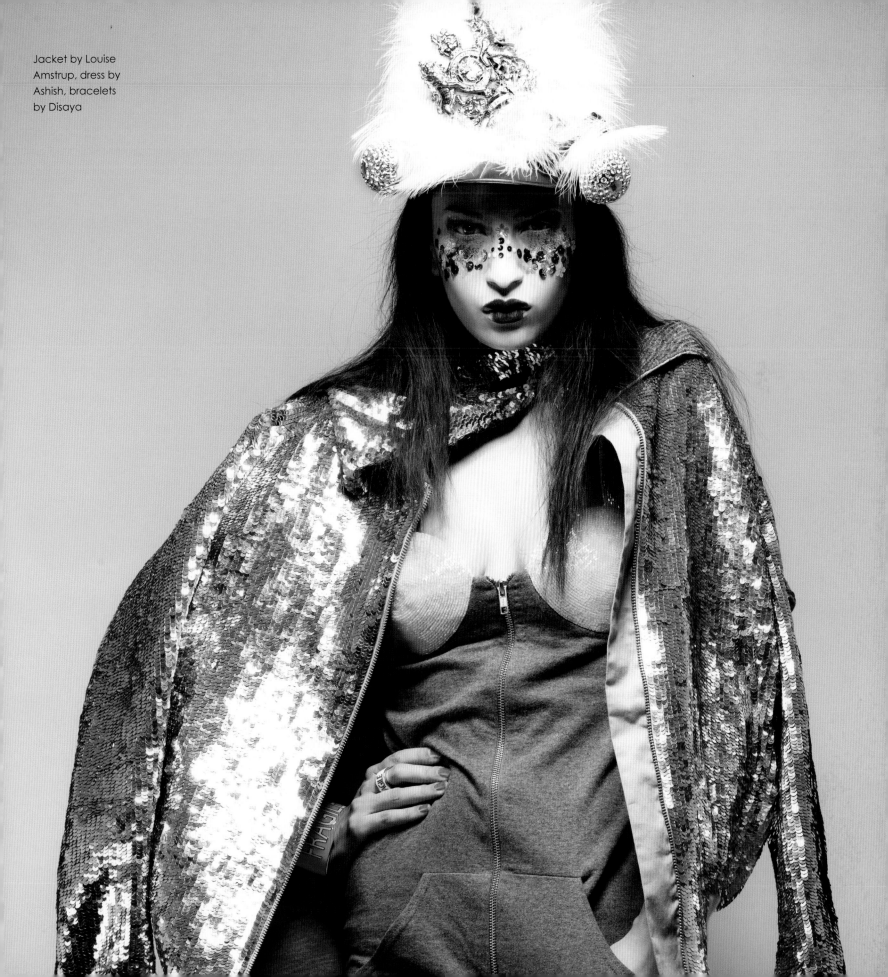

Jacket by Louise
Amstrup, dress by
Ashish, bracelets
by Disaya

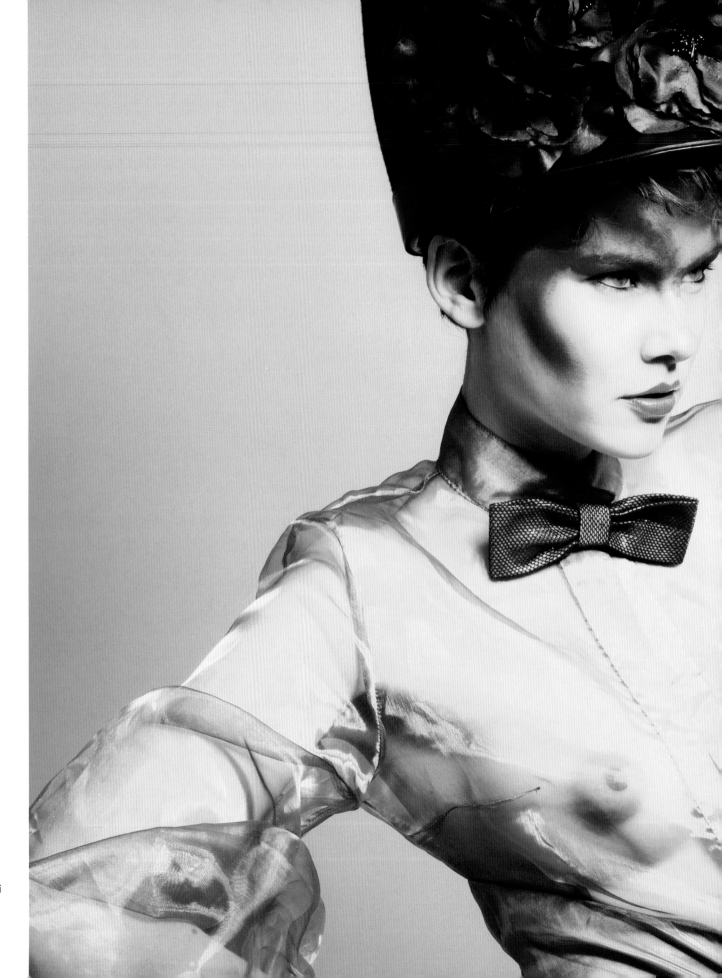

Photographer:
Camille Sanson
Makeup: Philippe
Miletto @ Terri Tanaka
Hair: Andrea Cossolari
Model: Erin @ Nevs

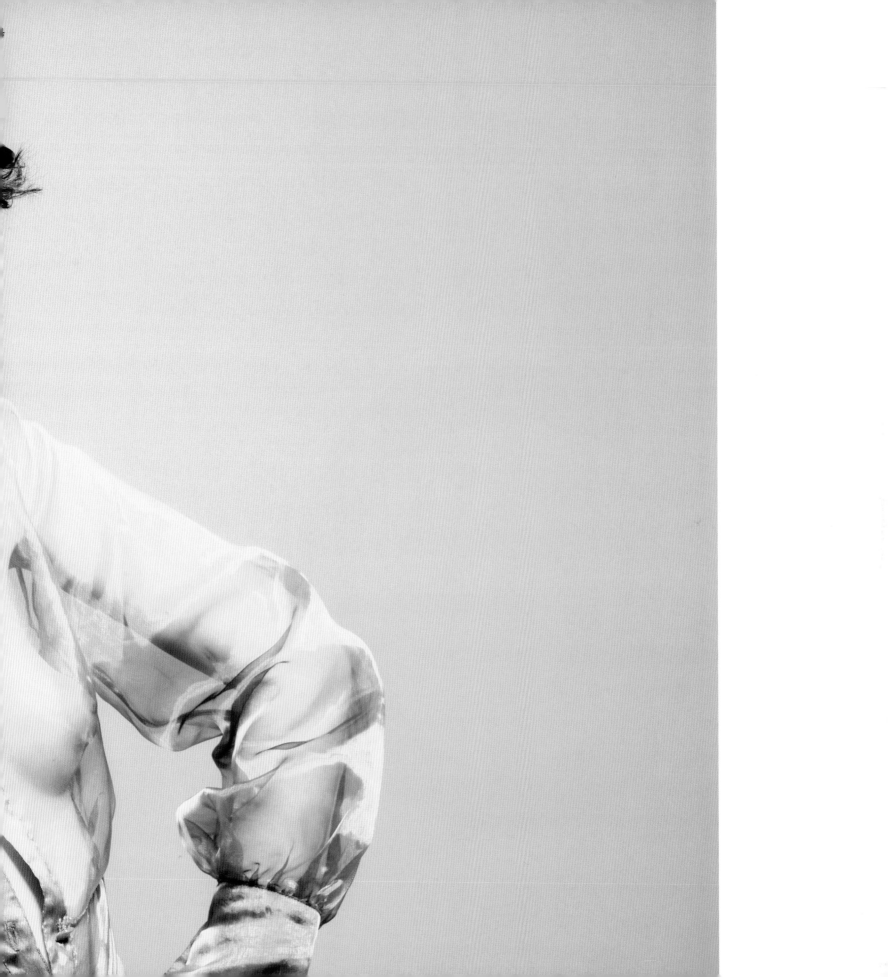

Nº5

The process of working from a fresh idea through to seeing the final story for an editorial piece is always exciting. Even though you have a vision in your head, sometimes the outcome may not be what you expected, due to many factors. You may run out of time because of unexpected challenges, which can slow the day down, so it is important the team is there for support and you must be prepared to be able to offer alternative ideas on the day. With careful planning, you tend to end up with something far better than you visualized to begin with.

Before the photo shoot, prep work will have started weeks before, from devising a theme to choosing the clothes, brands, makeup looks, lighting and sourcing the right location. These are all the key factors for an editorial shoot. You have an art director, makeup artist, hair stylist, fashion stylist, model and photographer.

Art in Motion: A Creative Brief for Clients

For a project working for Swarovski crystals, we came up with the idea of two modern, luxurious women, looking beautiful on a night out and enjoying a lavish lifestyle surrounded by crystals.

The sets were designed and sketched out with possible scenes. In order to successfully convey the luxury branding behind the advertisement, the location chosen to support it was the exclusive hotel No. 5 Cavendish Square in London. All the rooms were perfect for the setting we had envisaged – dark and decadent – and the props tied in perfectly with each room. All the props had been covered by hand in crystals, and took most of the day to set up. The model had been selected at an earlier stage through a casting and speaking process with the model agency. It is important for a model to have the right character and look for a shoot.

Makeup for this shoot was used to create a look that was timelessly elegant and groomed. The model's features were quite soft and delicate, so in order to make her look stronger, the eyebrows were groomed with an eyebrow gel and, once dried, lightened with full-coverage foundation. The eyes were contoured and defined with a mixture of cream and matte eyeshadows. Lips were natural matte to begin with and then darkened with a stronger colour to emphasize the change of scene and model. The model's hair was left down to work with all the hats and kept well groomed with a 1940s air of elegance. The lighting was moody, but had a lot of reflection from the garments and the crystals were brightened and enhanced by post-production retouching.

"The story was about a young woman who arrives in London and checks herself in to the boutique No.5 Cavendish Square Hotel for the night. Having been stood up by her date, she decides to have a wild night of her own. We wanted to achieve a sense of opulence and indulgence, and where possible use Swarovski crystals. We spent four days crystallizing fruit, champagne bottles, bowls, eggs and chocolate, applying each 3-mm crystal by hand. A tight budget meant we had to draw on every creative resource to get as much sumptuous fabric and as many crystals to dress the bedroom, bathroom and club. 'Breakfast in Bed' was when the beautiful girl wakes up… has a bath… and goes back to a bed of lush black velvet and liquid gold fabric to find a huge, ornate silver tray bursting with treats of Swarovski crystal eggs, apples, pomegranates and pears; cherries piled high on crystal ice cubes, crystal bowls of strawberries dusted with crystal sugar dust, a crystallized cake stand piled high with Lauderée macaroons in pinks and blues and gold, fine china tea cups, goldplated spoons in a bowl of crystal sugar cubes, a wondrous sparkling feast for the eyes, a glittering start to the day."

Misty Buckley, Set Designer

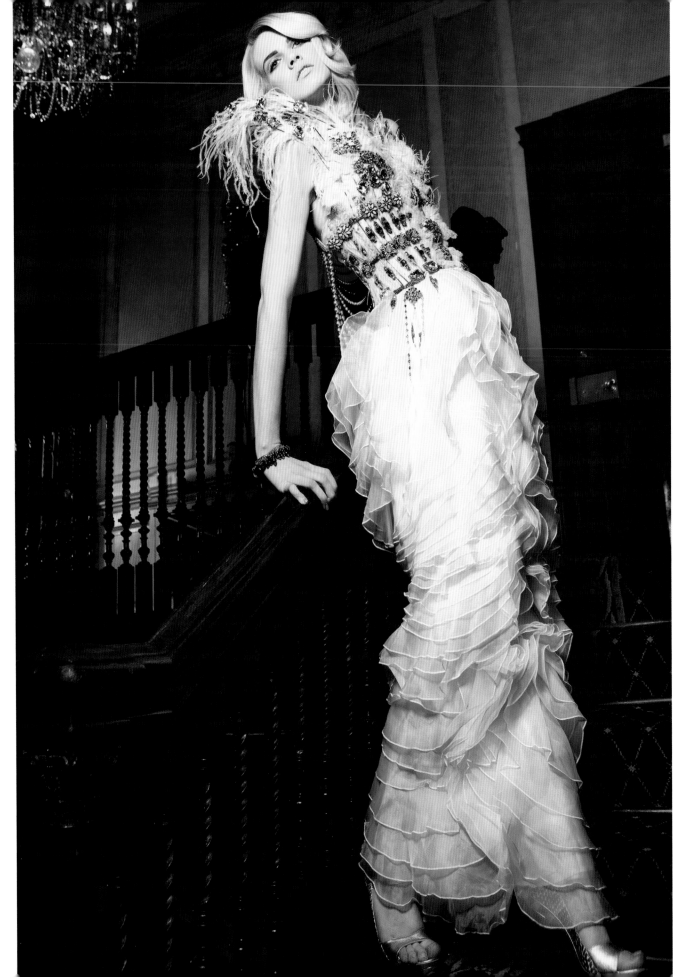

Photographer: Camille Sanson **Makeup:** Lan Nguyen using MAC and Swarovski **Hair:** Marc Eastlake using Bumble & Bumble
Stylist: Shyla Hassan
Set Designer: Misty Buckley **Set Assistants:** Richard Olivieri and Reggie Matheson
Model: Birgit @ First Model Management
Photography Assistants: Pau Cegarra and Laurie Noble **Makeup Assistant:** Karla Barchieri @ AOFM Agency.
Special thanks to Mark Whittle at No. 5.
Dress by Ruth Tavardos worn with a corset by Erickson Beamon for Swarovski Runway Rocks, shoes by Gil Carvalho

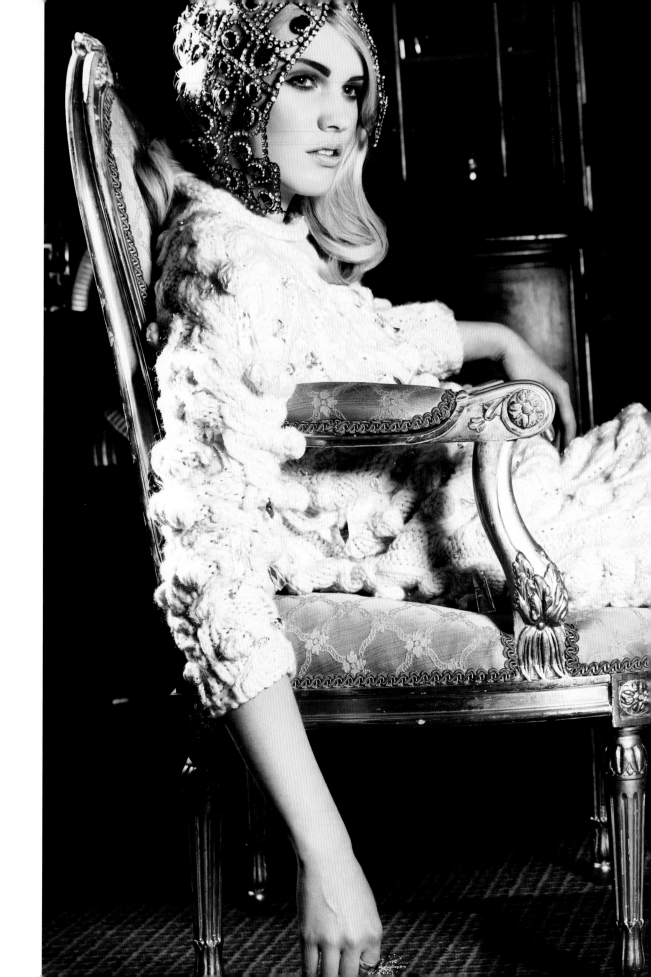

Hat by Danilo for
Swarovski Runway
Rocks, jumper by
Jullien Macdonald
for Swarovski Runway
Rocks, shoes by
Gil Carvalho, jewellery
by Erickson Beamon

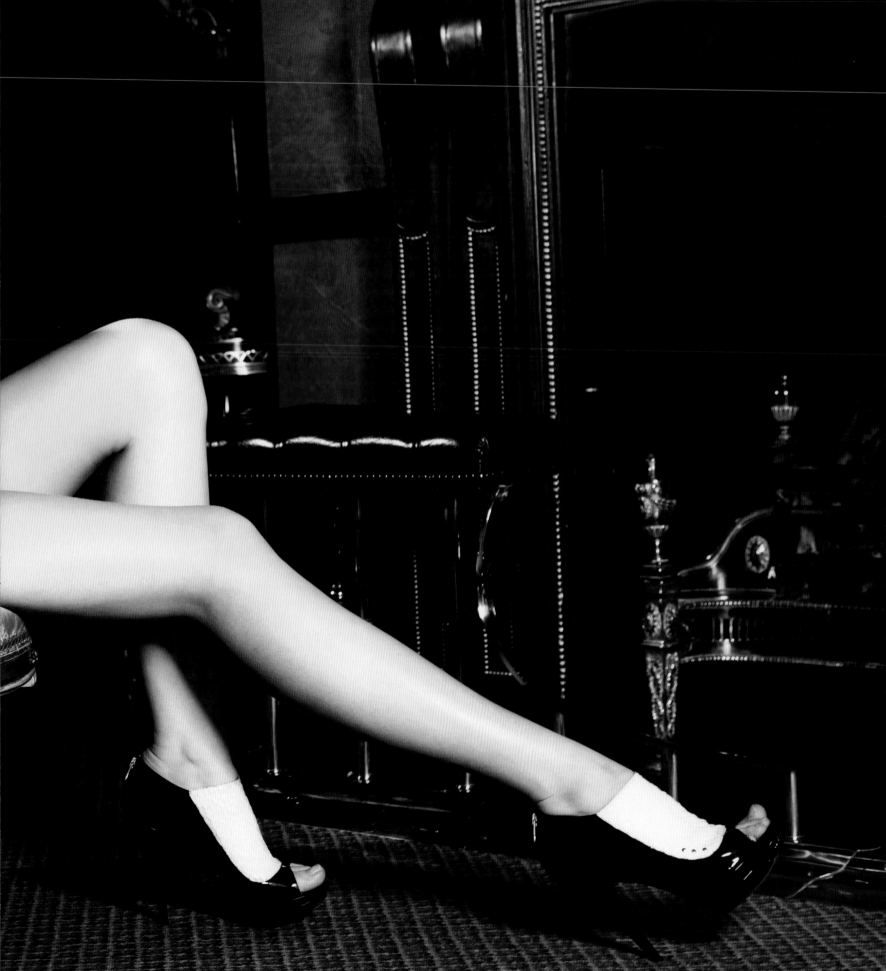

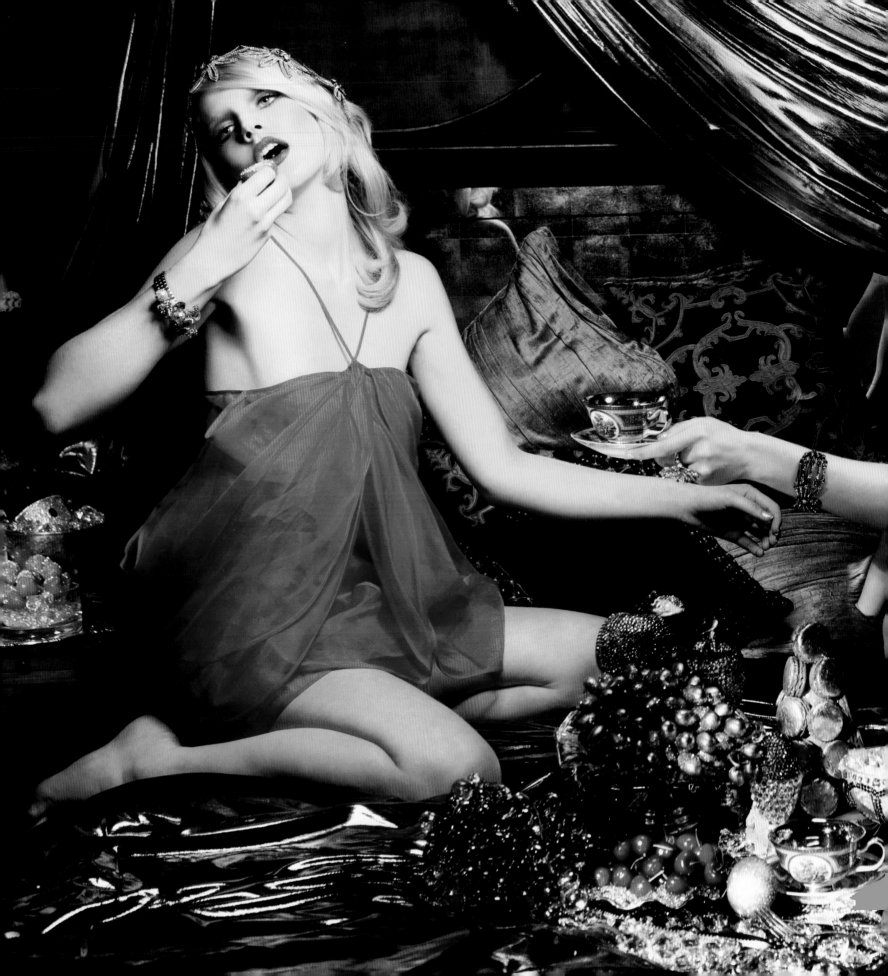

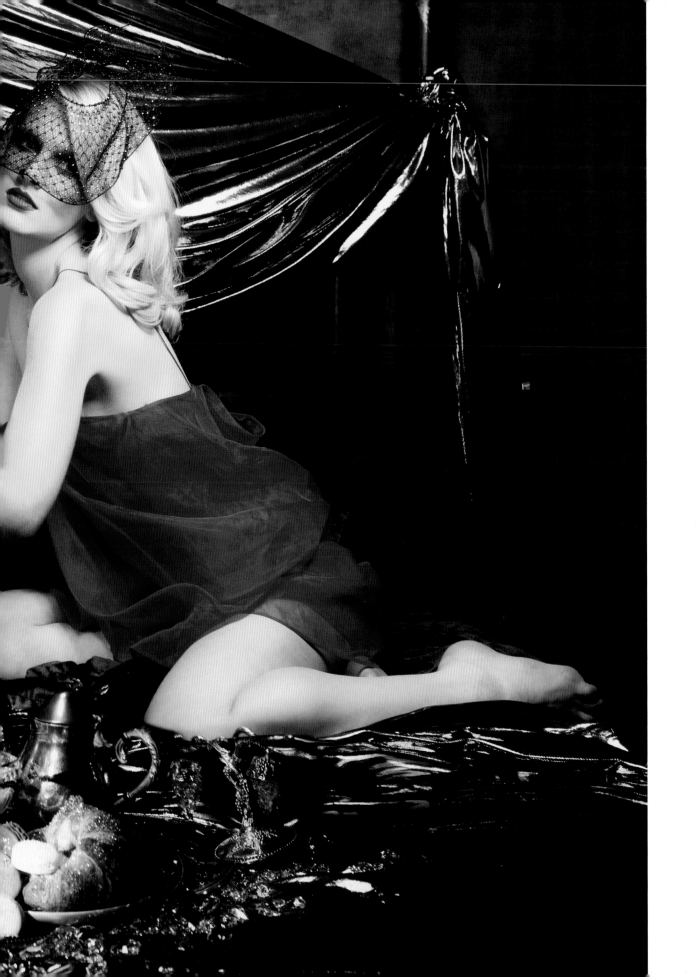

Red dress by Ruth
Tarvydas, head band
by Louis Marriette,
head piece by Philip
Treacy for Swarovski
Runway Rocks,
jewellery by
Erickson Beamon

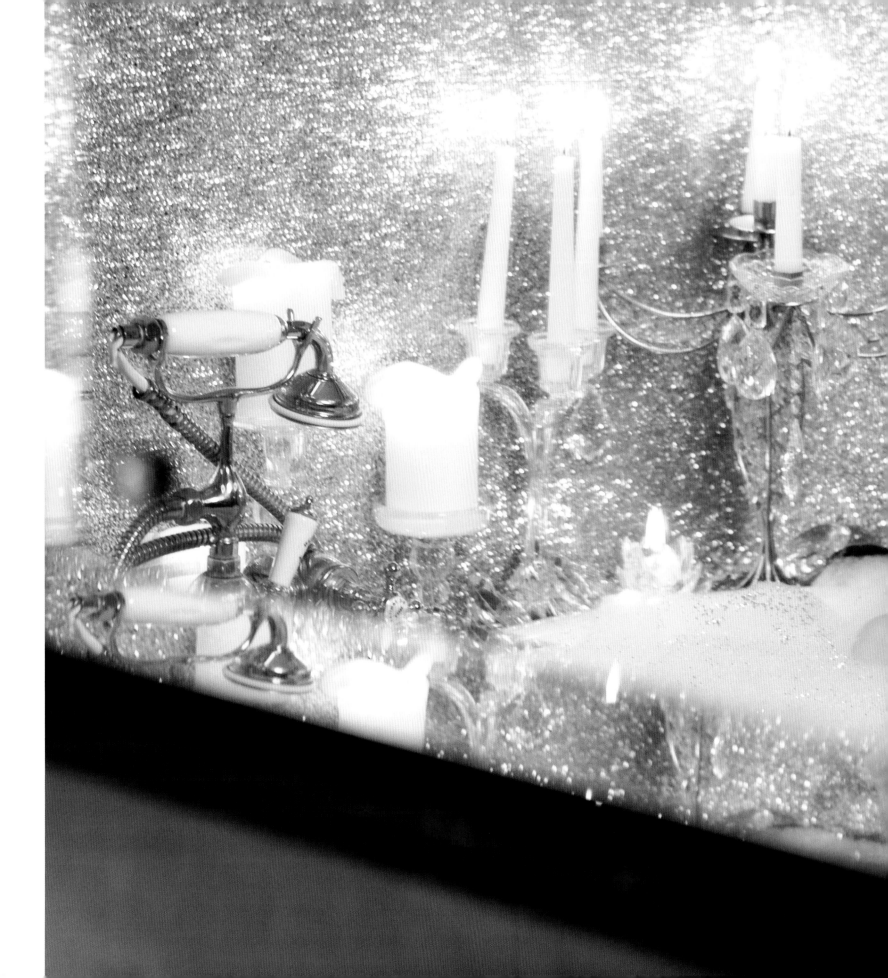

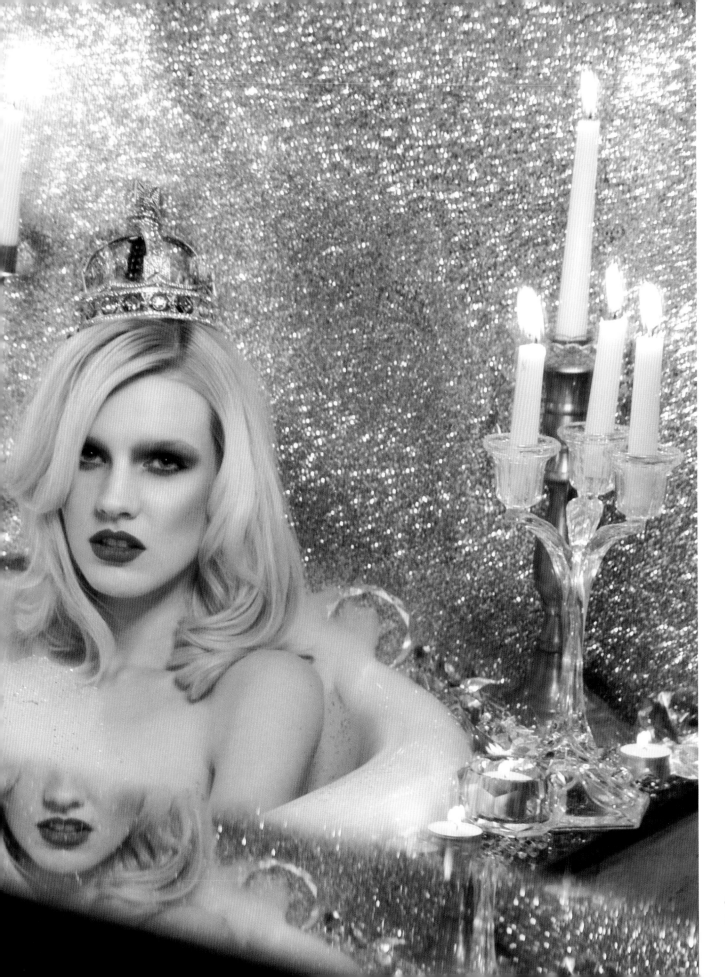

Crown by
Louis Marriette

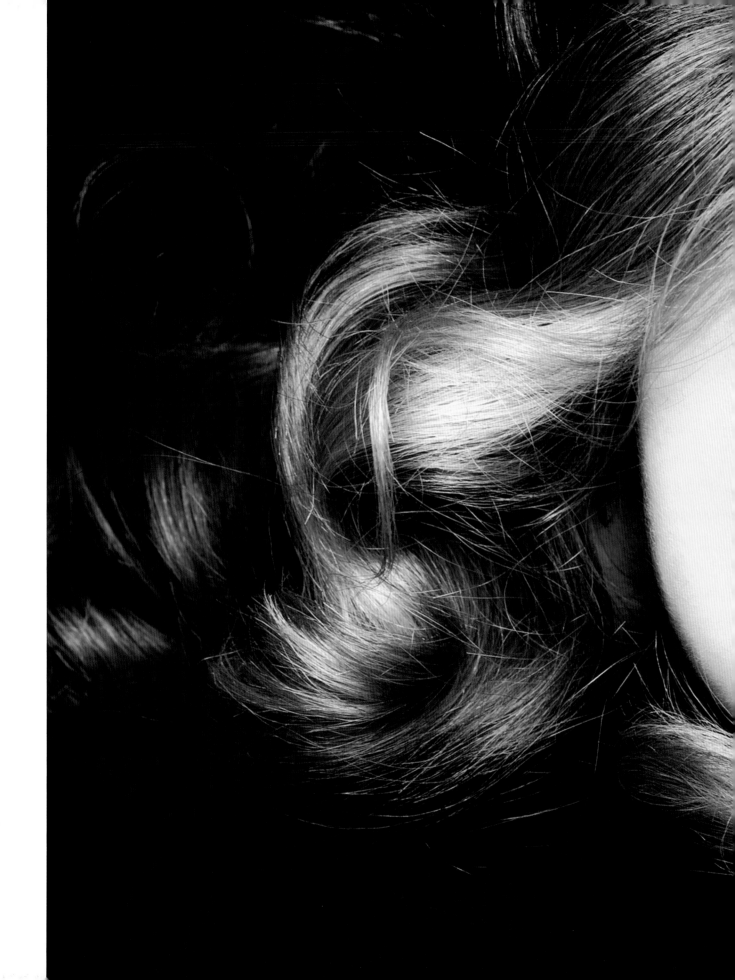

BEAUTY *EDITORIAL*

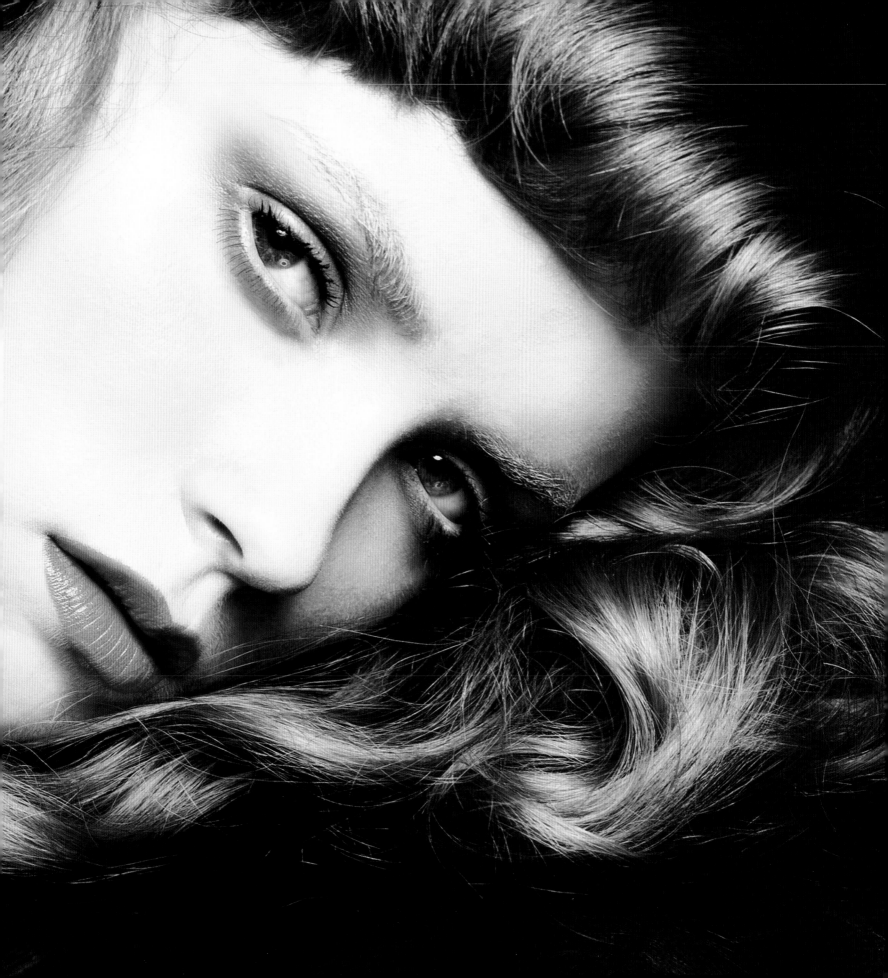

POST-PRODUCTION

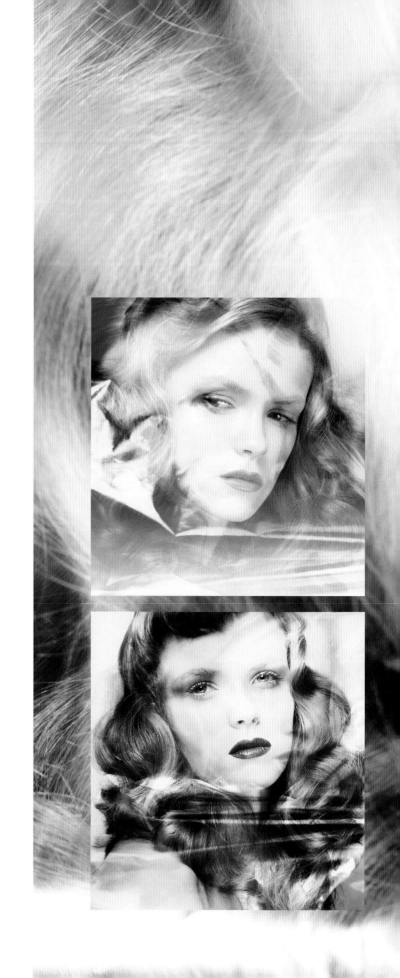

A photographer's job extends beyond standing behind the lens and capturing the shots. When everyone's working day is over, the photographer must start work on the post-production process. Post-production is the general term used to describe the process of turning the raw shots from the camera on the day of the photo shoot into the polished, glossy images we see in magazines.

The first step of post-production is the selection of images. Often hundreds of images are taken in any one day of shooting, so narrowing down to the best is a big job, often with only miniscule differences between the shots. The team, including hair, makeup and styling, may help with this process and narrow them down to a smaller number of potential final images. Once the final images are selected, retouching is carried out to perfect and tweak the images.

Retouching Images

A widely standardized practice in magazines and advertising campaigns, in order to smooth out wrinkles, fine lines, lumps, bumps and blemishes, retouching can also be used to stretch out models, slim models down and remove cellulite, which can result in an unrealistic picture of beauty.

Retouching allows small errors to be rectified, for example, if a model's lipstick has faded in one corner, a few stray hairs need to be removed or there are clumps of mascara. Knowing photographs can be retouched can sometimes lead to sloppiness, as some makeup artists may feel they do not have to work hard to perfect their makeup application.

Although the responsibility of retouching belongs to the photographer, the makeup artist should review the images, make sure they are happy with them and that they are projecting their work, and ensure that the makeup has not been completely altered.

Photographer: Camille Sanson **Makeup:** Lan Nguyen using Dior
Hair: Kuni Kohzaki
Model: Danielle Foster

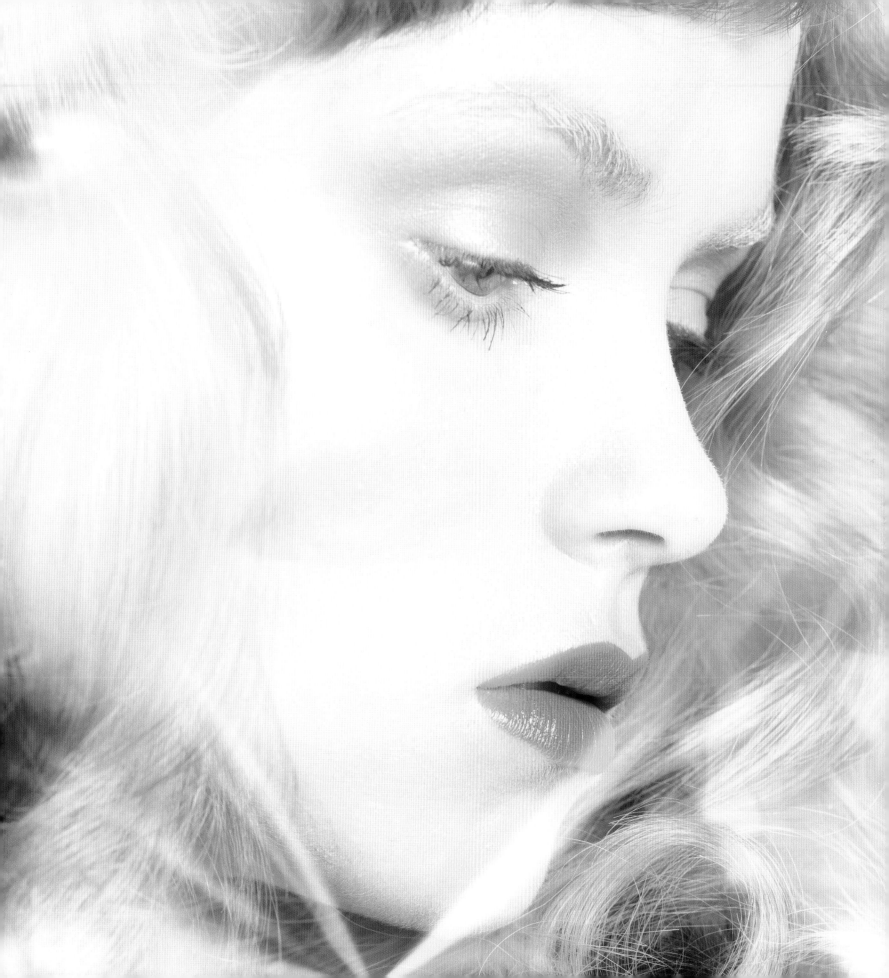

ADVERTISING

Makeup artists are almost always used in advertising. An example of this may be the appearance of sweat on the brow of a sportsman in a Nike commercial, or the pigtails on a little girl in a toy advert.

From the commercial advertisements you see on television to billboard posters; a makeup artist was needed on the shoot to ensure the people being photographed or filmed were looking their best. The look or type of makeup a makeup artist will do on the "talent" (how the model or actor is referred to on set) is very job-specific. The makeup look not only has to fit in with the story of the advertisement, but also has to be appropriate for the product it is advertising.

Photographer:
Camille Sanson
Makeup: Lan Nguyen
using Lancôme
Hair: Marc Eastlake
Stylist: Shyla Hassan
Model: Sabrina @ Next
Dress by Bora Aksu

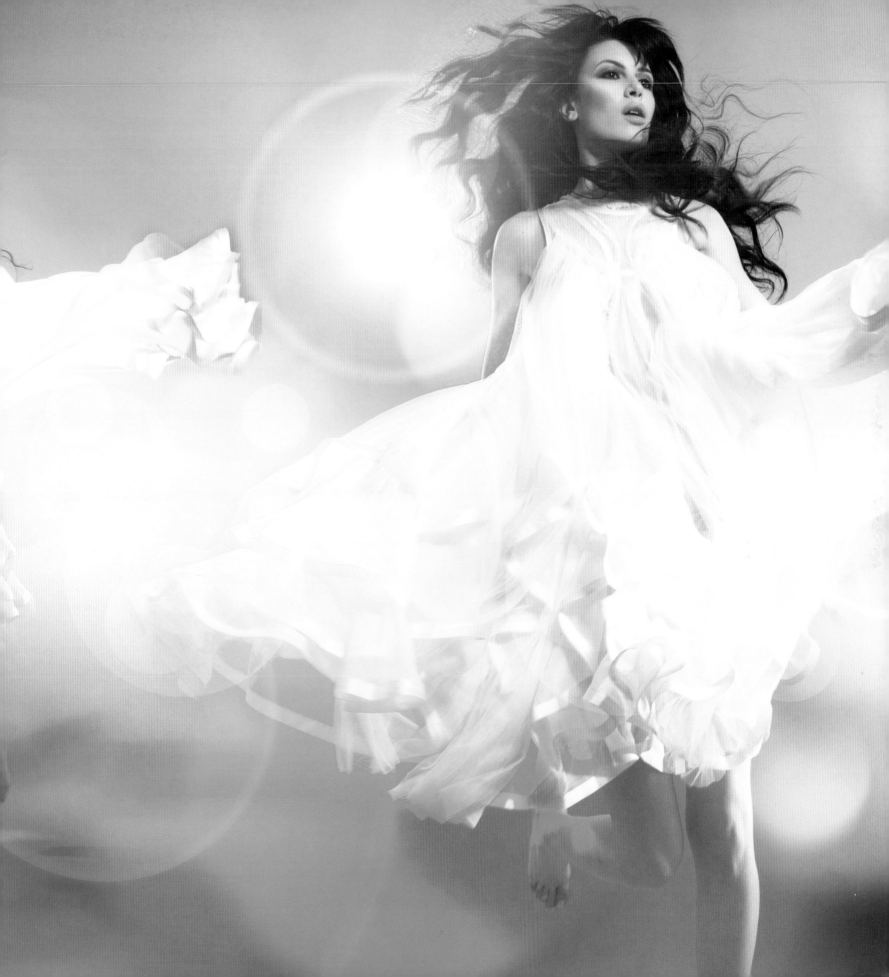

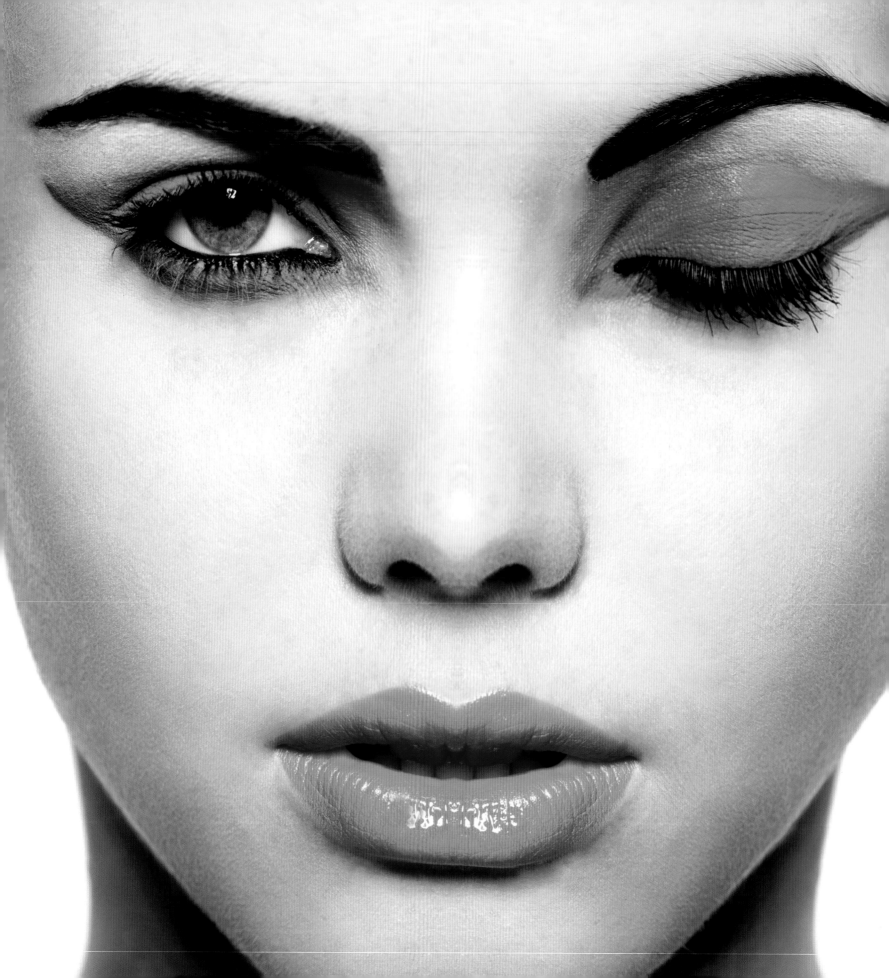

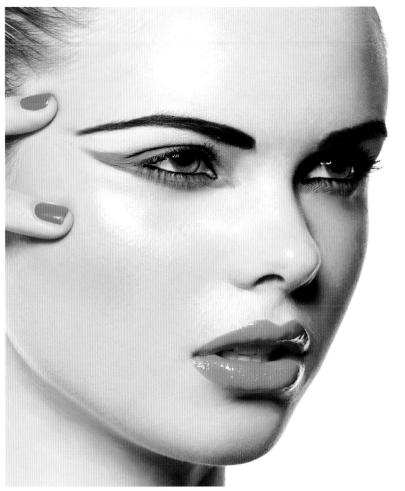
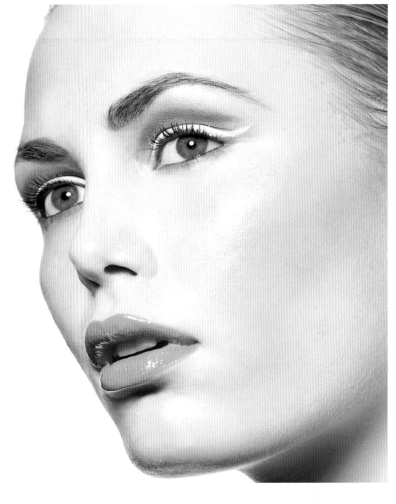

COLOUR EFFECTS

Here we created the look for an advertisement for Kryolan professional makeup. Before designing the look, we had to research the brand: who are the customers and what does the brand stand for? Kryolan is a specialized manufacturer of professional makeup serving theatre, film and television; they also supply products to the beauty sector.

In advertising work, you have to be prepared with a wide variety of looks in case the original idea does not work. Ask yourself whether the look should be natural or strong, and what products should be used to promote the brand. Having the right balance of looks to attract a customer is important, as is knowing what is going to make the image stand out. Sometimes campaigns are modified to make the image stand out more, but it is important that the look shown is its truest form, according to the aims of the brand.

Once the skin had been prepped, a full-coverage foundation was used to create a flawless airbrushed effect. Cheeks were kept soft, with contoured with a brightly coloured blush, applied lightly. For the eyes, strongly pigmented greasepaints were used, placing colours in sections on the eyelid – the colour was kept in solid blocks to show the true colour pigments. Blending at the sockets with another bright colour opened up the eye shape. The eye was all about strong, graphic colours, rather than smudging, which would have made it look softer.

Eyebrows were filled in to create a modern twist and to help give a more graphic feel. Lips were also blocked in with a solid colour to complement the rest of the look. Adding highly coloured gloss to the lips helped to keep it looking modern. Various colours were used in different areas of the face, and the model was shot at different angles to provide variation.

Photographer:
Catherine Harbour
Makeup: Lan Nguyen
using Kryolan
Models: Gabriele
D and Larissa H @
Premier

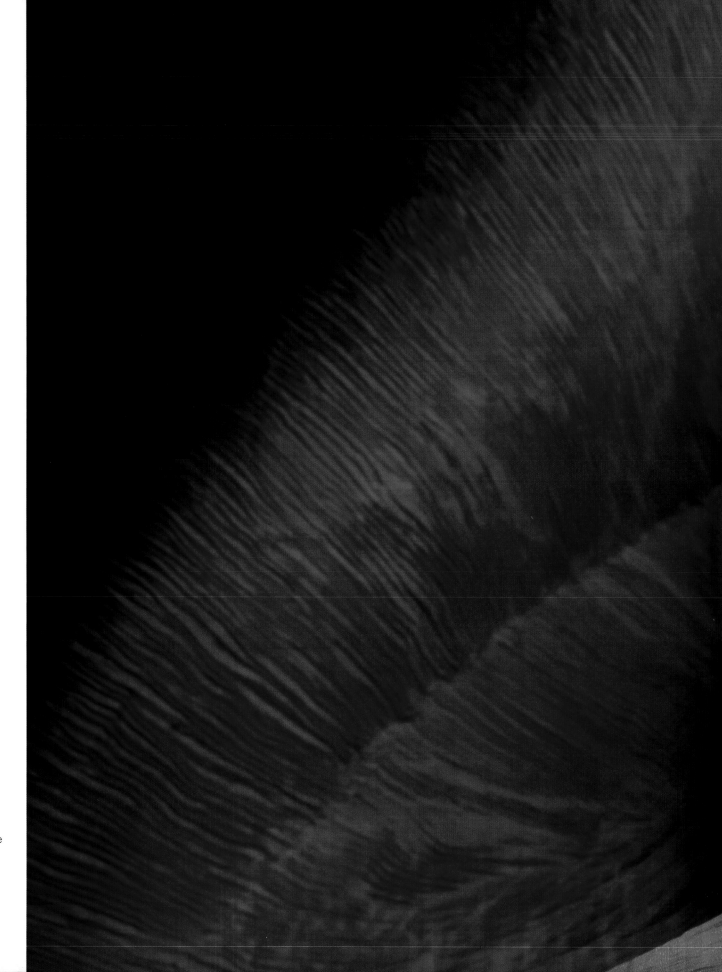

Photographer: Camille Sanson **Makeup:** Lan Nguyen using Shu Uemura **Hair:** Andrea Cassolari **Model:** Hannah @ Next

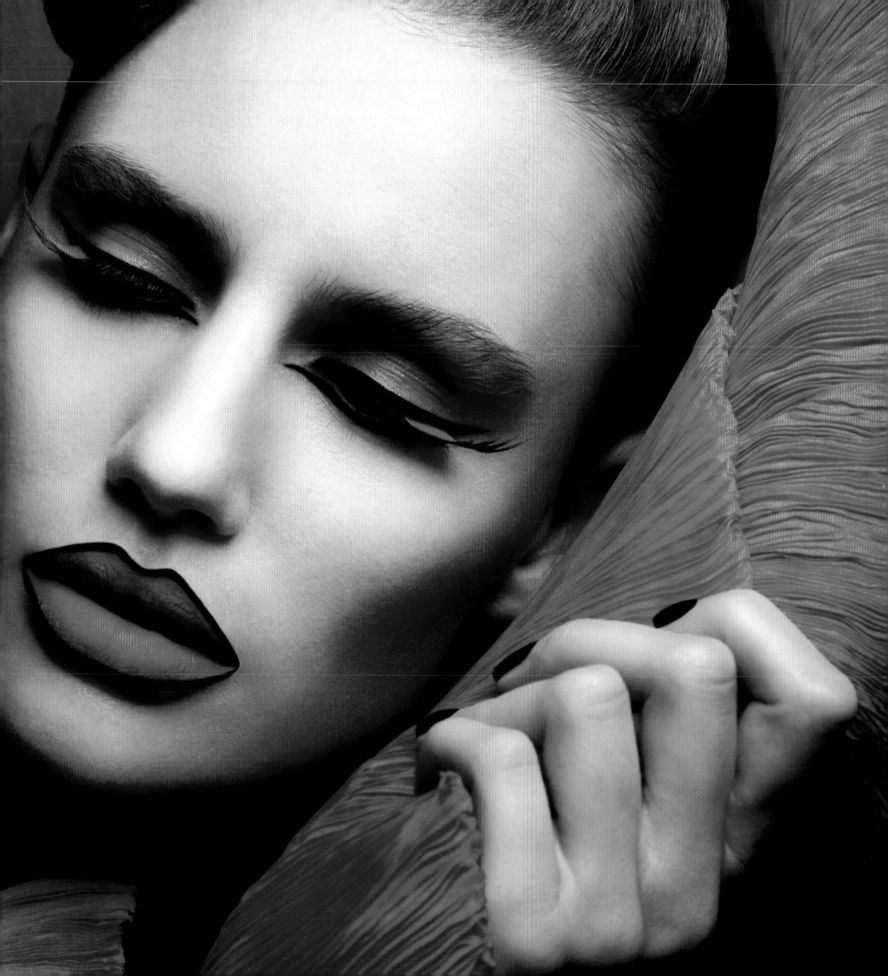

CONCEPTUAL

Avant-garde makeup is as infinite as one's imagination. It is all about pushing the boundaries and encourages you to think outside the box. Prime examples of this type of makeup look can often be seen on the catwalk at Paris couture fashion week. Designers John Galliano and Jean-Paul Gaultier are two of the leading trendsetters of this look.

Many designers showcase their work to demonstrate their individuality and cutting-edge values. Often, their clothes are considered to be more like wearable art. Therefore, the makeup designs that complement the clothes can also be seen as quirky and beautiful art works.

The concept of the makeup designs, the colours used and how and where the makeup is applied, can influence the commercial market, too, and inspire the creation of new makeup products. Brands including Charles Fox, MAC and Shu Uemura are constantly developing interesting makeup ideas for professional artists. This constant stream of development means there is no limit to what you can create.

The catwalk shows also inspire the future trends and avant-garde editorials in magazines. High fashion magazines such as *Numero*, *10*, *Dazed & Confused* and *Pop* are just some of the many that take inspiration from the catwalk and create their own images for the public domain. They ultimately feed the makeup and styling world with even more creative imagery and new looks.

Photographer: Zoe Barling **Makeup:** Sandra Cooke using MAC **Hair:** Natasha Mygdal using Bumble & Bumble **Model:** Alex C @ IMG

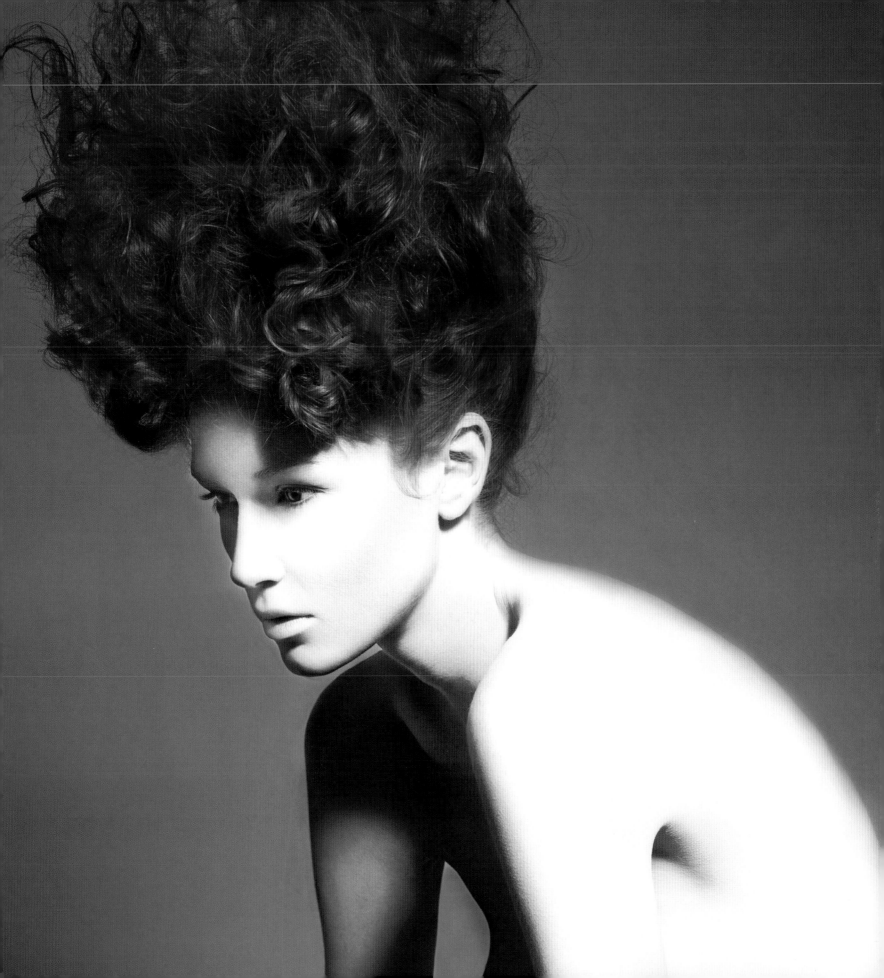

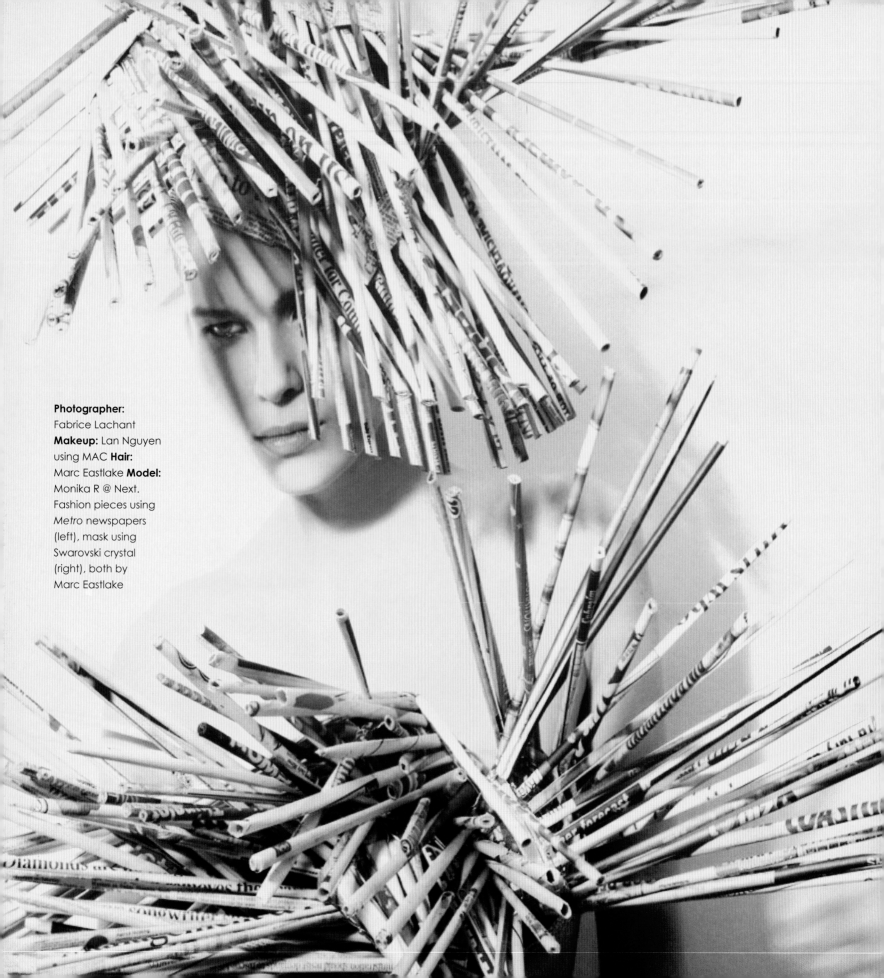

Photographer:
Fabrice Lachant
Makeup: Lan Nguyen
using MAC **Hair:**
Marc Eastlake **Model:**
Monika R @ Next.
Fashion pieces using
Metro newspapers
(left), mask using
Swarovski crystal
(right), both by
Marc Eastlake

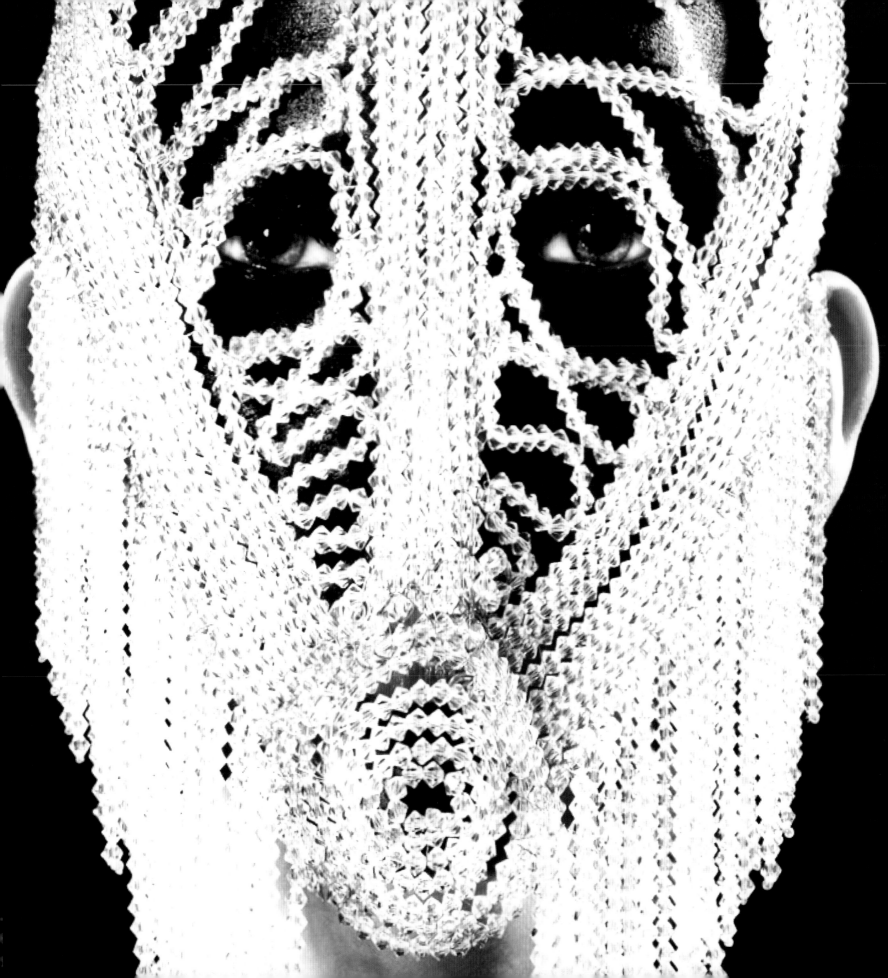

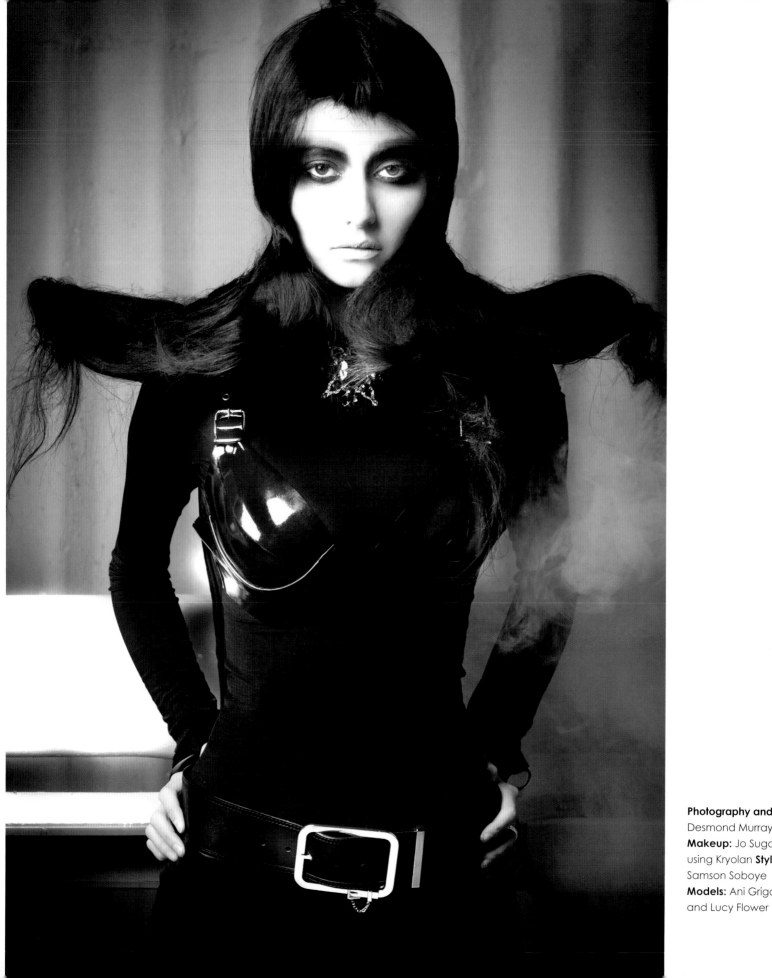

Photography and Hair:
Desmond Murray
Makeup: Jo Sugar
using Kryolan **Stylist:**
Samson Soboye
Models: Ani Grigorian
and Lucy Flower

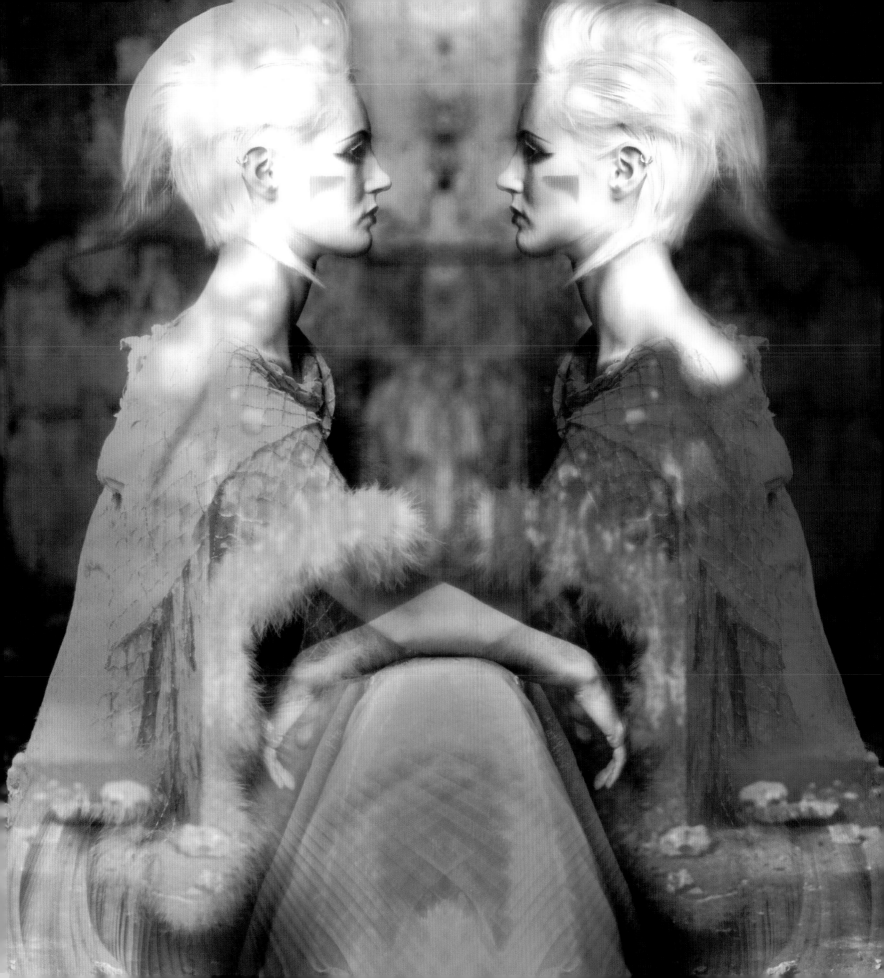

Photographer:
Catherine Harbour
Makeup: Philippe
Miletto using MAC
Hair: Andrea Cassolari
Model: Iliza @ Next

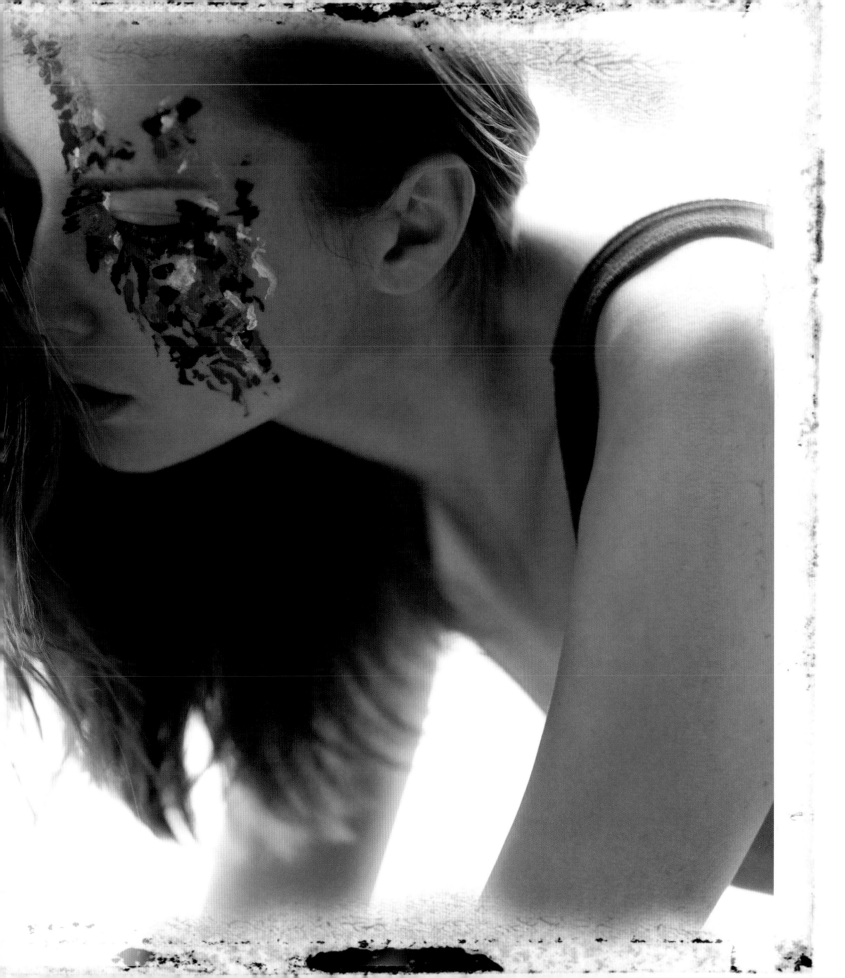

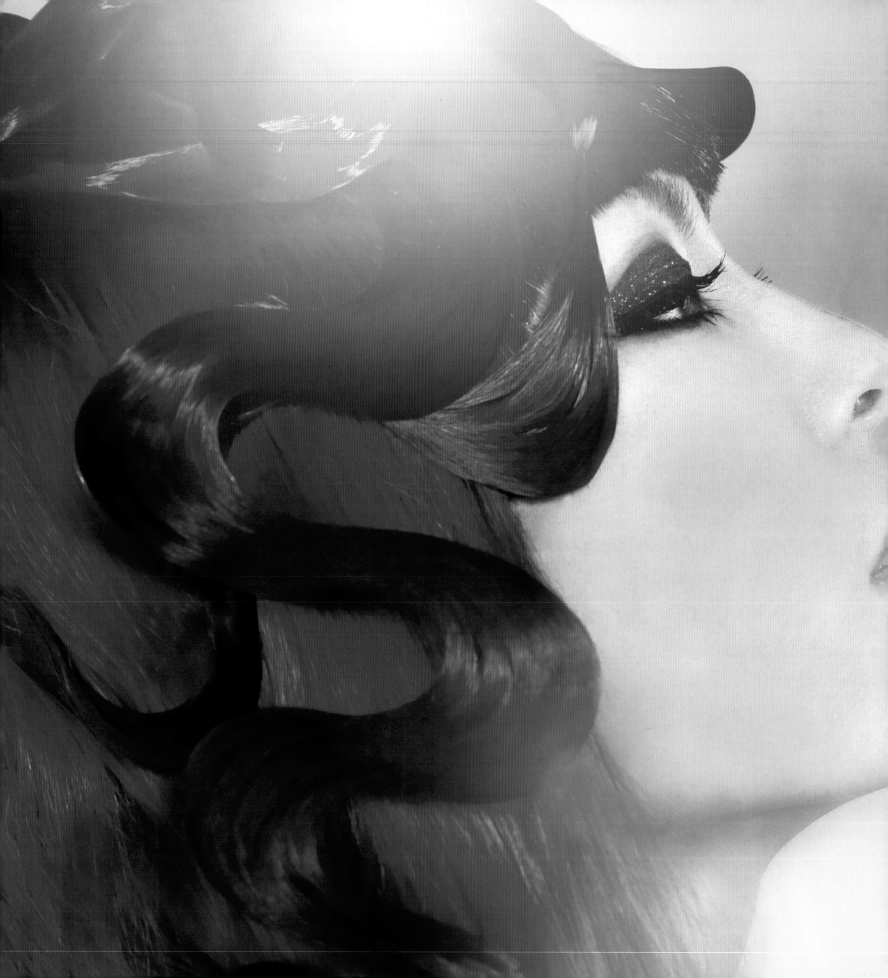

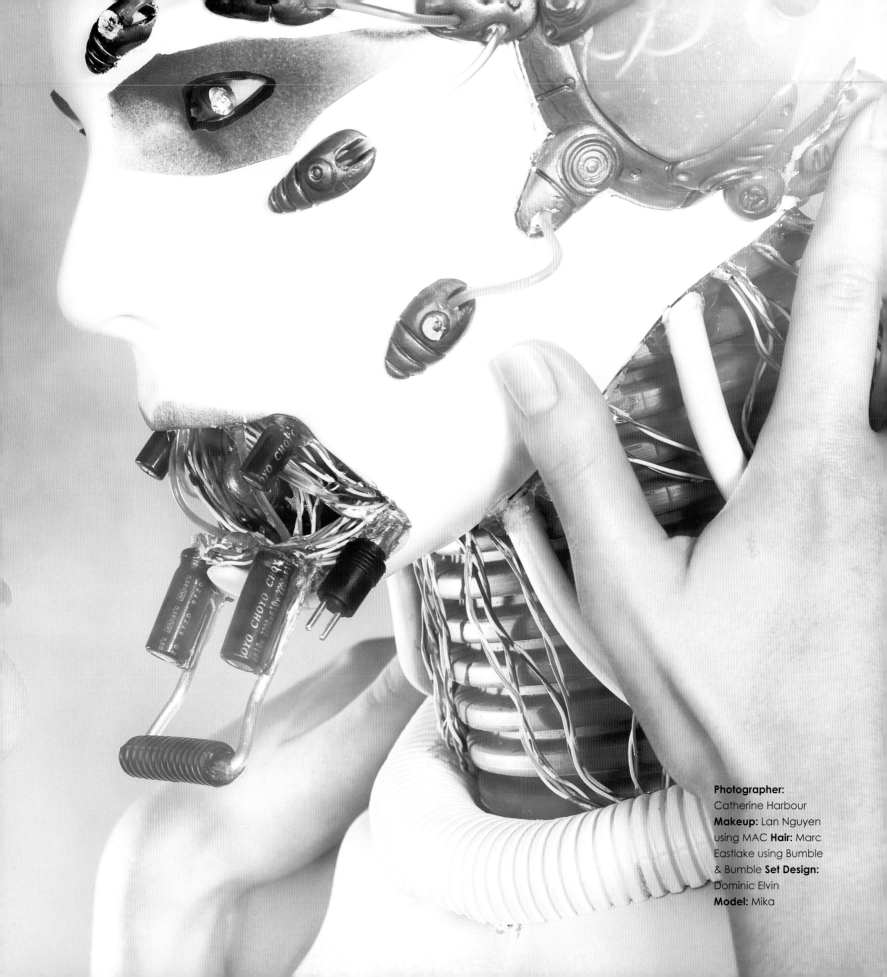

Photographer:
Catherine Harbour
Makeup: Lan Nguyen
using MAC **Hair:** Marc
Eastlake using Bumble
& Bumble **Set Design:**
Dominic Elvin
Model: Mika

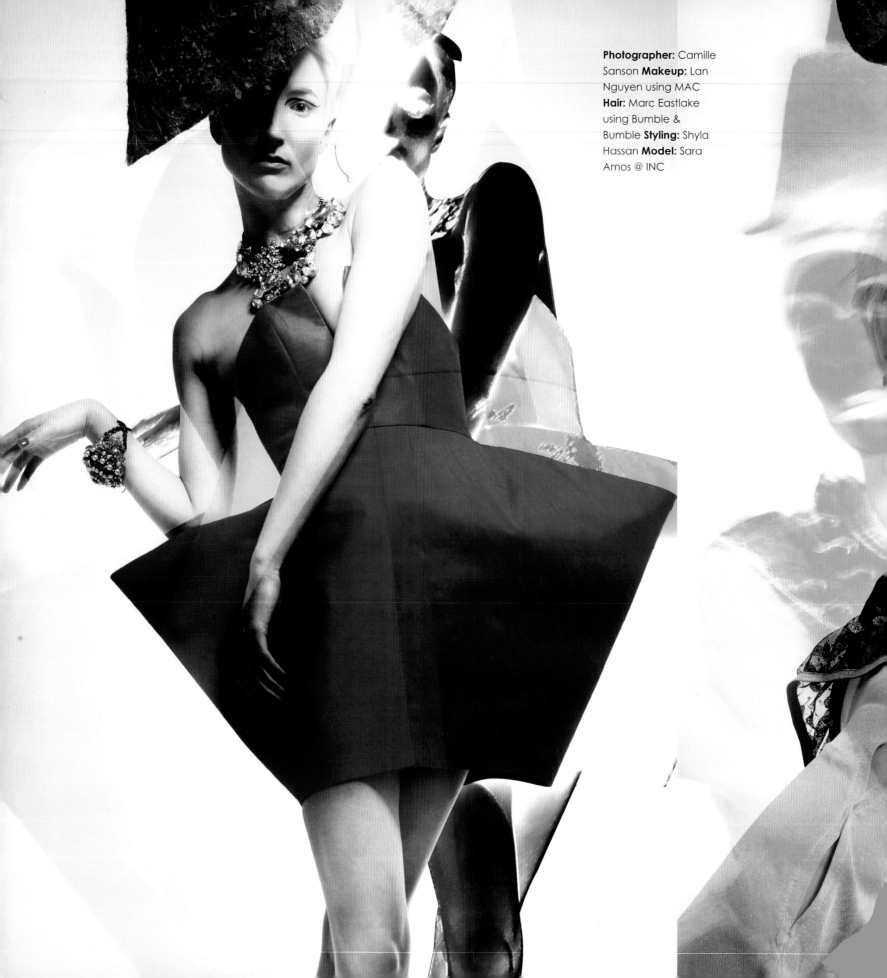

Photographer: Camille Sanson **Makeup:** Lan Nguyen using MAC **Hair:** Marc Eastlake using Bumble & Bumble **Styling:** Shyla Hassan **Model:** Sara Amos @ INC

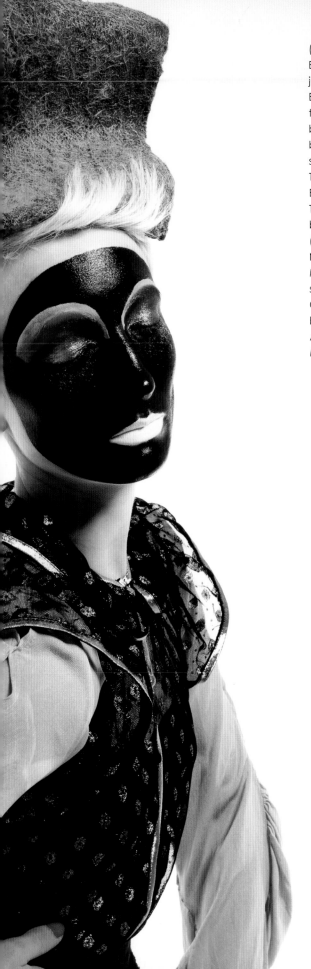

(far left) Blue dress by Bernard Chandran, jewellery by Erickson Beamon. (left) Mesh top with gold spots by Topshop, peach blouse, stylist's own, skirt by William Tempest. (right top) Black dress by William Tempest, jewellery by Erickson Beamon. (right bottom) Navy waistcoat by Modernist, cream shorts by Bernard Chandran, jewellery by Erickson Beamon. All head pieces by Marc Eastlake

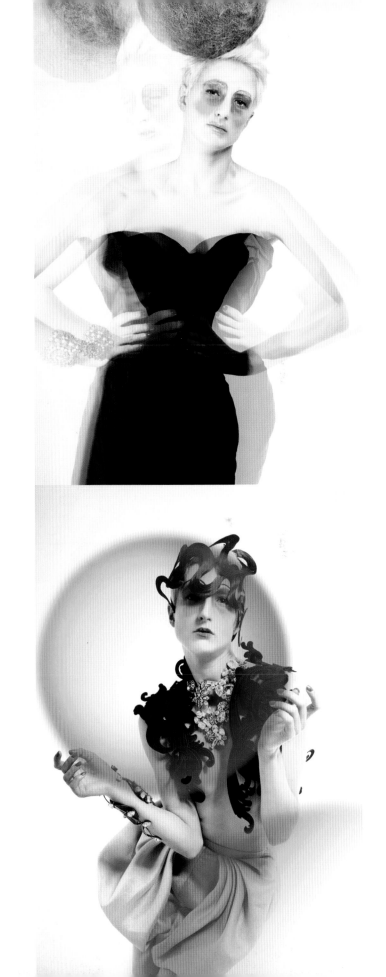

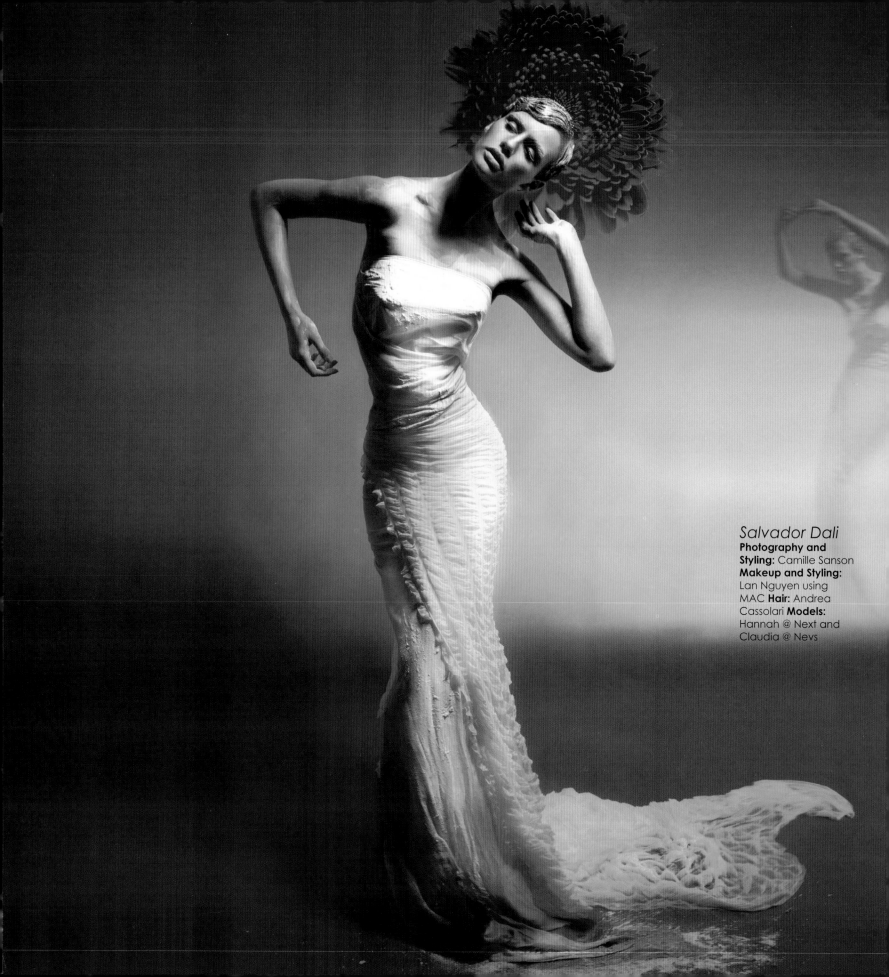

Salvador Dali
Photography and Styling: Camille Sanson
Makeup and Styling: Lan Nguyen using MAC **Hair:** Andrea Cassolari **Models:** Hannah @ Next and Claudia @ Nevs

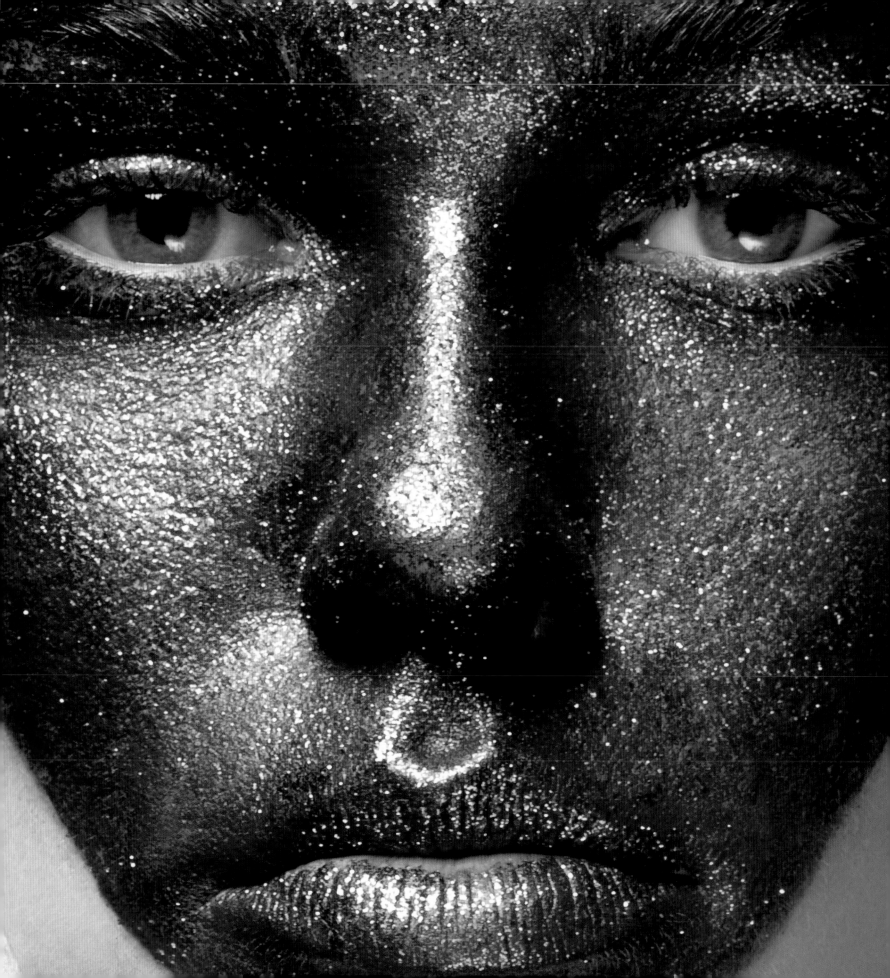

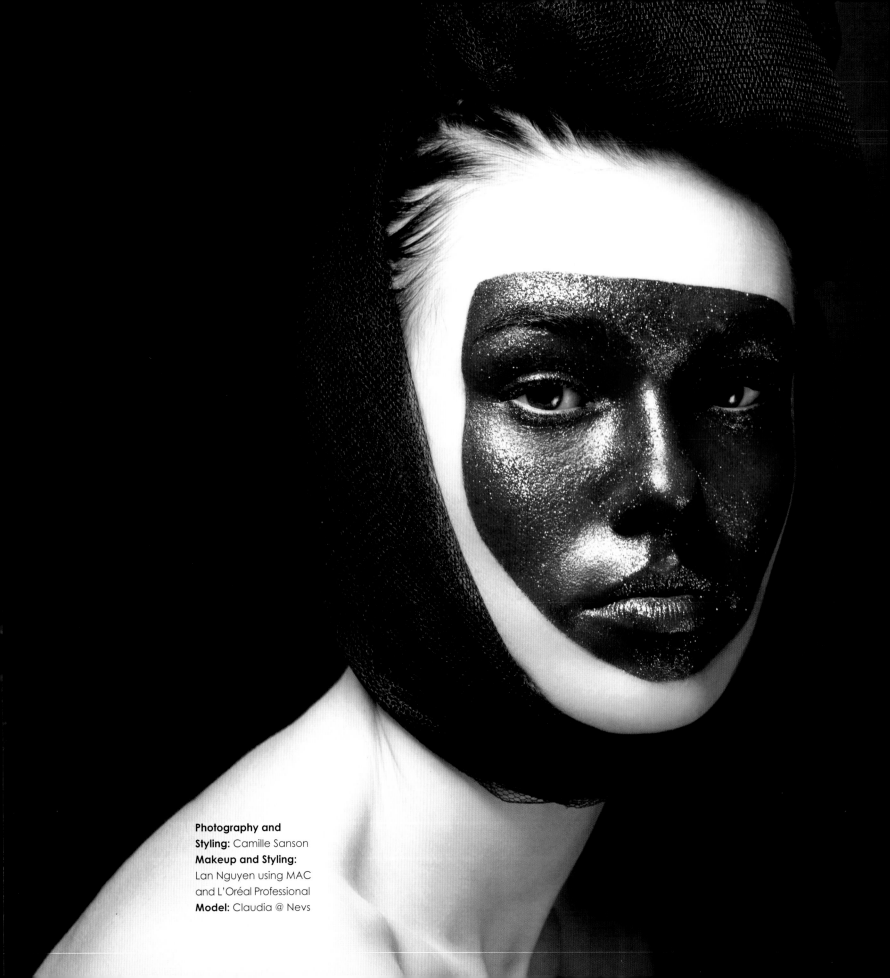

Photography and Styling: Camille Sanson
Makeup and Styling: Lan Nguyen using MAC and L'Oréal Professional
Model: Claudia @ Nevs

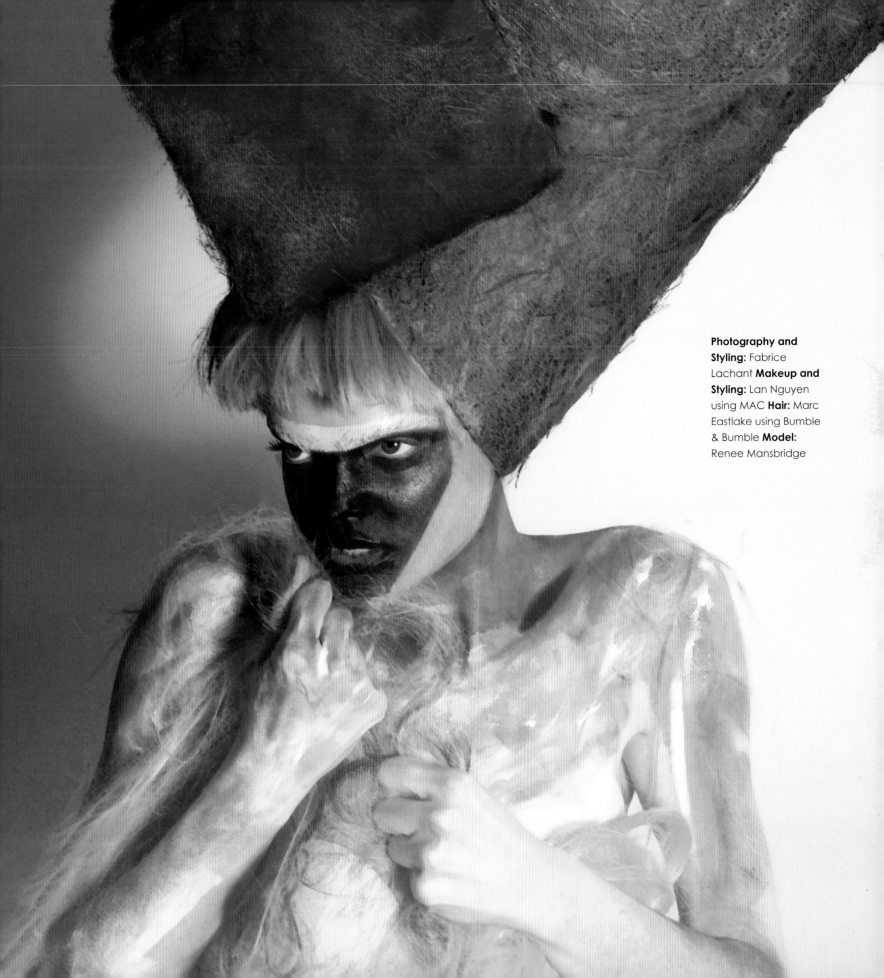

Photography and Styling: Fabrice Lachant **Makeup and Styling:** Lan Nguyen using MAC **Hair:** Marc Eastlake using Bumble & Bumble **Model:** Renee Mansbridge

BODY ART

Body decoration is one of the oldest forms of art. Historically it has been a tradition of many ancient tribes across the globe, using materials such as coloured clay and charcoal. It has now entered the mainstream and is used in mediums such as ad campaigns, album covers and fashion shows.

Body painting is an increasingly competitive industry. It is important to have the skills needed before taking on any professional jobs, as good-quality work is not something you can easily achieve without plenty of practise. Know the paint's limitations as well as your own. Work a design through with a client from their initial concept to the final approved design. This way, you will be sure that what you are producing is according to plan, you will feel confident about the job and, ultimately, you will produce an amazing piece of art. To get repeat business, remember that you are only ever as good as your last job.

Techniques and Equipment

There are two main techniques: brush and sponge painting and airbrushing. It is easiest to start with a few simple brushes, sponges and face paints. A basic kit should consist of primary and neutral colours, such as black, white, red, yellow and blue. You do not want to spend all your time mixing, so green, purple, pink, orange, grey and brown are also handy staples.

Brushes

When choosing brushes look for ones with dense bristles, as they will cause less streaking. Below is a selection of basic brushes to have in your tool kit.

- A brush with a curved edge for smooth lines.
- A flat, straight-edged brush to create well-defined lines.
- A large flat brush that is at least 5cm (2in) wide to cover large areas of the body quickly.
- A medium-sized flat-edged brush.
- A small, flat-edged brush, square to rectangular in shape, to create straight lines and crisp edges.
- A fine-pointed brush for detailed work, and for working from a thick line to a thin one.
- Face painting sponges to blend colours on the body, cover underwear in paint and get into awkward areas, especially around the eye area.

Using Paints

Body paints are made according to stringent guidelines – they are non-toxic and non-allergic. Because the paints are activated with water, you will find that when you try to layer your colours they may start to blend into one another. For example, if you paint white detail over a black background, you will quickly find that the bright white turns grey. It is much easier to cover a lighter colour with a darker colour than the other way around. When necessary however, fix your base coat with a fixing spray or strong-hold hairspray. This will help eliminate blending problems.

Airbrushing

It is expensive buying all the necessary equipment, but there are other tools that can be used to create dramatic effects when a paintbrush is not enough. An airbrushing kit consists of a compressor, an airbrush gun and special paints. Airbrushing is an extremely useful skill to have when you work on jobs that require a lot of stencilling and when you want very softly blended highlights and shadows.

To use an airbrush gun you push down on the trigger to start the airflow and pull back on the trigger to release the paint. The lighter you press it, the softer the airflow, and the more you pull back, the more paint is released.

Once you get used to the way the gun works you will be able to create anything from a line as thin as a hair to a smooth, perfectly blended background. Practise on cheap canvases and with acrylic paint to build your skills. When you can, practise on a model so you can get used to working on a living, breathing and sometimes moving canvas.

Working with Models

When planning your work, think about the order in which you want to cover the body. When body paint is dry it is relatively touch-proof, but it will smudge easily if rubbed. It is often best, if working with a female model, to cover their breasts first so she feels less exposed and more comfortable.

Leave certain areas of the body such as the mouth, hands and bottom, clean or without detail initially, as most detailed body paints will take between three to six hours to be completed and during this time, your model will probably need to sit down, eat, drink and use the bathroom.

Some models will struggle having to stand up for such long periods of time without moving, so make sure you have sugary snacks and drinks on hand to keep energy levels up. Some might not want to drink a lot of water because they are worried about needing to visit the toilet and smudging the paint, so be sure to reassure them that it is a lot easier to clean up smudged paint than having to clean off an entire section because your model has fainted!

Photographer: George Kuchler
Makeup: Carolyn Roper using MAC
Models: Carolyn Roper and Craig Tracy

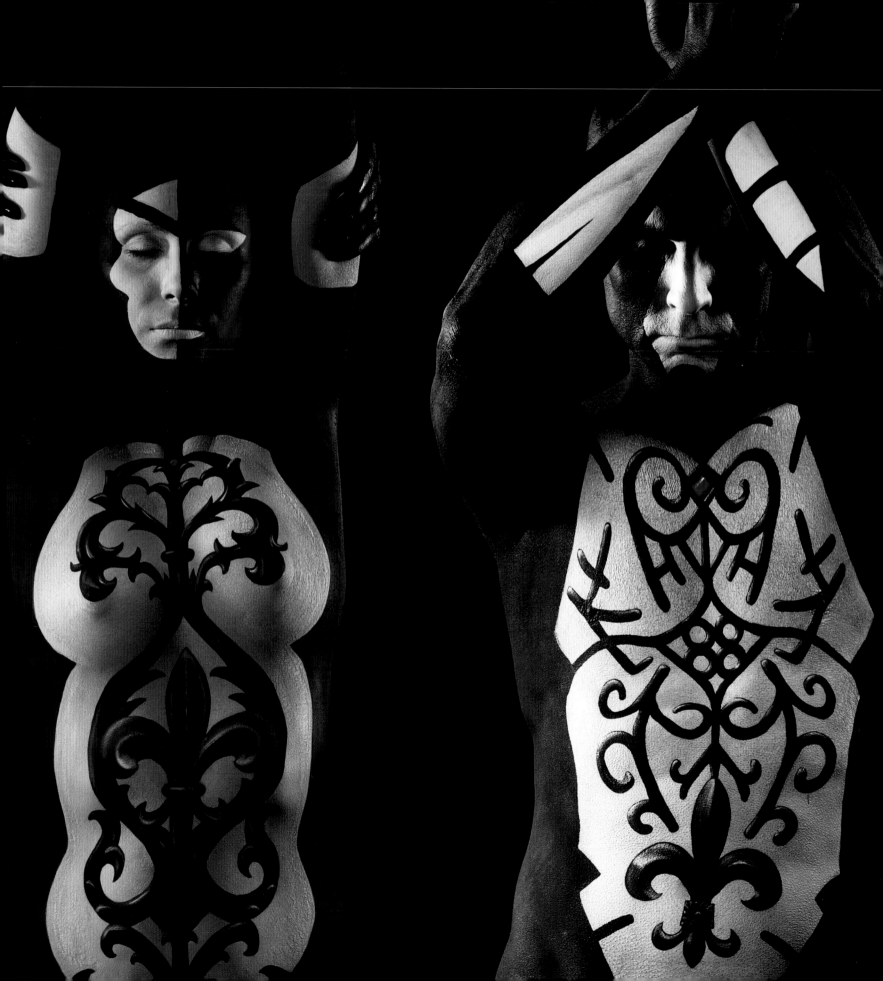

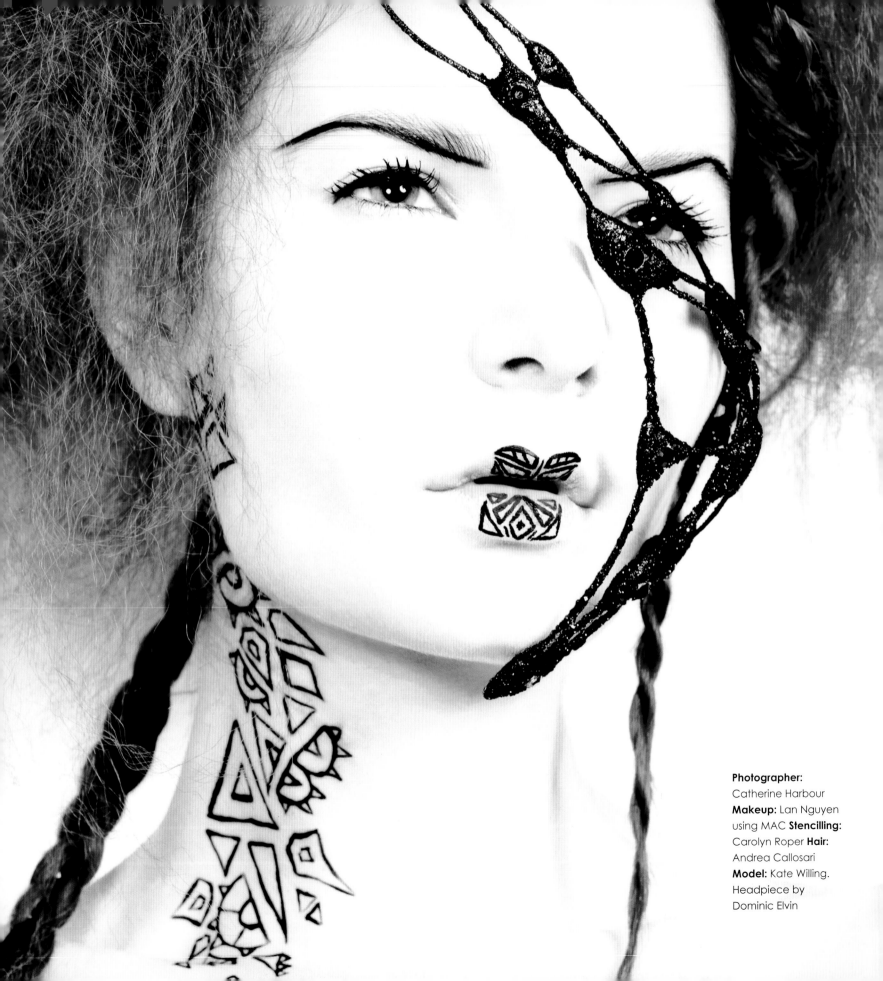

Photographer:
Catherine Harbour
Makeup: Lan Nguyen
using MAC **Stencilling:**
Carolyn Roper **Hair:**
Andrea Callosari
Model: Kate Willing.
Headpiece by
Dominic Elvin

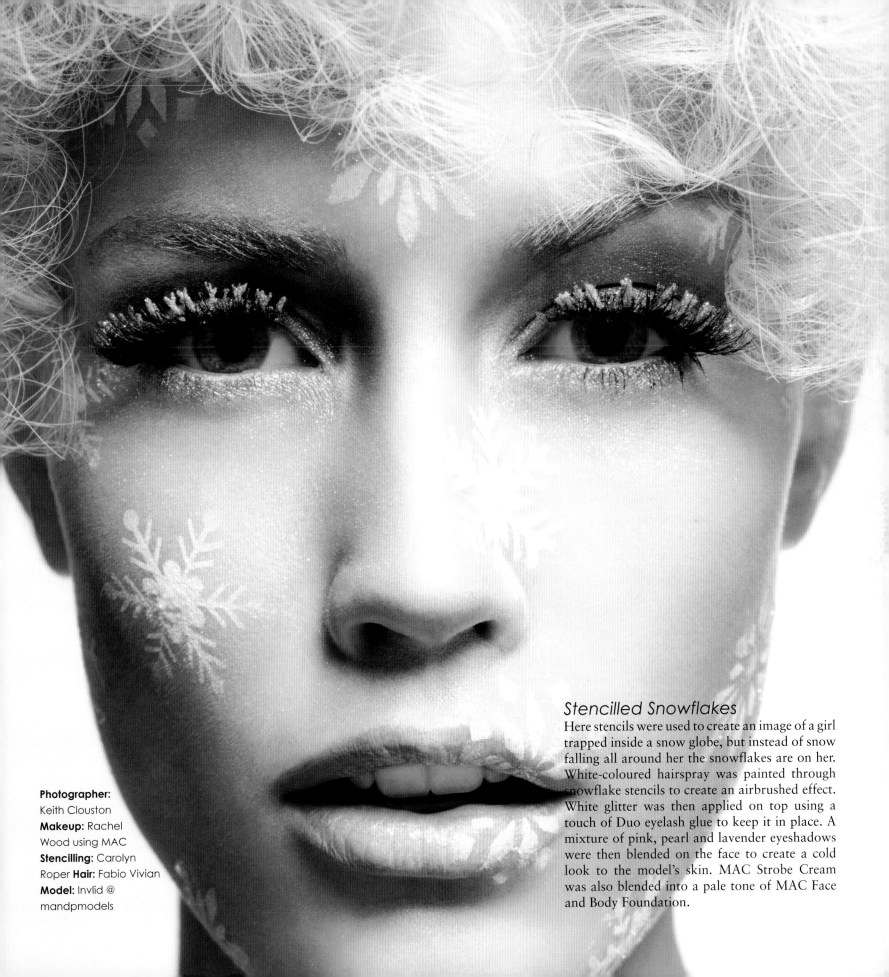

Stencilled Snowflakes

Here stencils were used to create an image of a girl trapped inside a snow globe, but instead of snow falling all around her the snowflakes are on her. White-coloured hairspray was painted through snowflake stencils to create an airbrushed effect. White glitter was then applied on top using a touch of Duo eyelash glue to keep it in place. A mixture of pink, pearl and lavender eyeshadows were then blended on the face to create a cold look to the model's skin. MAC Strobe Cream was also blended into a pale tone of MAC Face and Body Foundation.

Photographer:
Keith Clouston
Makeup: Rachel
Wood using MAC
Stencilling: Carolyn
Roper **Hair:** Fabio Vivian
Model: Invlid @
mandpmodels

CONCEPTUAL BODY PAINTING

This is a modern interpretation of an Art Deco-style painting, inspired by the work of Polish artist Tamara de Lempicka. Taking the colours and main characters from some of the original paintings, the design was worked around the shape of the body.

The main design was created using Kryolan Aqua Colours and Airstream Airbrush paints, and is complemented by simple beauty makeup using pigments in the same shades as the paint. The fine lines that fan out around the two main figures were created using very fine glitter glue, also used to frame the face. Crystals around the eyes and cheekbones, attached with hydro-mastic body glue, completed the design. The steps below can be adapted for any body-art idea.

1 When planning the design, remember that your main canvas areas are the front and back of the torso, so this is where you want to position your main details. The arms and legs are a good place to get creative with colour blending.

2 Always start by painting the basic outline of the design in the colour that relates to the finished image. This makes it easier to work out where different colours start and finish and makes blocking in the rest of the colours less confusing.

3 Once the base lines are drawn, start putting on the base coat. Always mix the paint to a really creamy consistency, as this will ensure the base coat doesn't streak. When the base coat is finished you can start to add the details.

4 Body paints sink into each other over time and will not look as vibrant, so it is important to start with the shadows and leave the highlights until the end. Adding a layer of sealant in between the base coat and your detail is the best way of minimizing colour corruption.

5 Airbrushing creates beautiful, soft highlights and shadows and is used at the end of the painting to create a real sense of depth.

Photographer: Lou Denim **Makeup:** Carolyn Roper using Kryolan **Model:** Femke @ Nevs

• To avoid tell-tale join marks, cover the largest areas, such as the chest and back, first and finish at the sides where joins will be far less noticeable to clients and photographers.

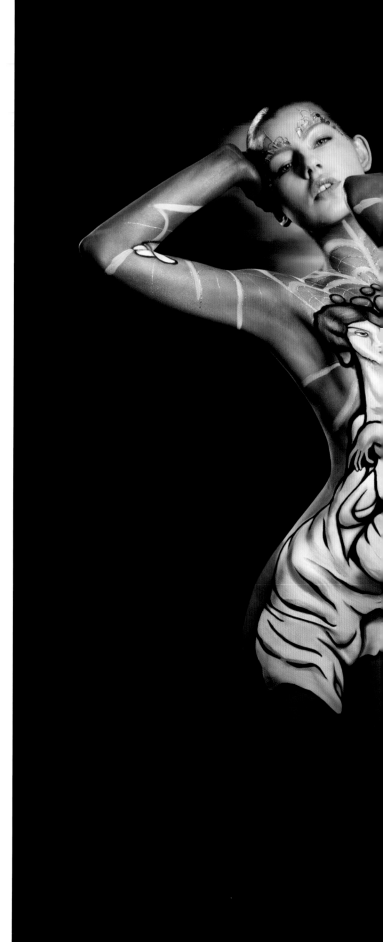

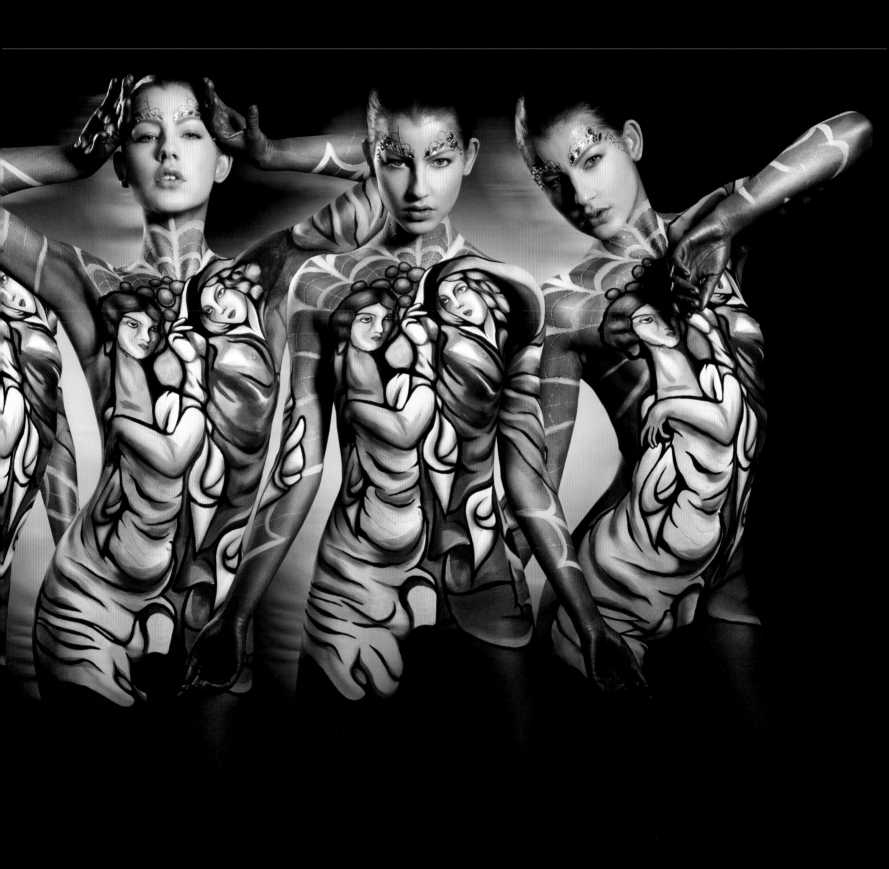

COLLABORATING

"Collaborating with makeup artists is always different, depending on what the brief is. For instance, when I am shooting for the British Hairdressing Awards, it is predominately about the hair, so the relationship is with a team of people and the mood board. The mood board will dictate the feeling of the whole shoot, ensuring the makeup artist, photographer, fashion stylist as well as the hairdresser are all singing from the same hymn sheet. Sometimes the hairdresser will know what they want from the makeup, other times they will not, so the makeup artist will have more input in the design of the makeup.

Sometimes, on a hair shoot, it may not be clear what is wanted with the makeup, so there will either be a prep day in advance or the team will arrive early and play with the makeup to see what works. This way there is plenty of scope for individual creativity and freedom.

Fashion shoots are totally different, especially if it is a test shoot. Everyone experiments and is pushing the boundaries in their own field, but the team comes together for the overall look – it is not just about one person, it is a collective effort.

When doing fashion shows, the focus is on the clothes. Before the show there will be a fitting where the head hair stylist and makeup artist create their looks on a model and present them to the designer to see if it works. If the designer is happy, then the heads go back to their teams and brief them with the look. This needs to be done very quickly, so there is very little time for prepping and often the hair and makeup is being done at the same time. The makeup artist needs to work in tandem with the hairdresser and vice versa.

When working with celebrities, they dictate their image so you have to liaise with makeup and styling. It is all about what the celebrity wants and creating an overall image, so you may be recreating a style they are known for rather than having creative input."

Desmond Murray, Celebrity Photographer and Hair Stylist

Photography and Hair: Desmond Murray
Makeup: Jo Sugar using Charles Fox
Model: Sophie Willing

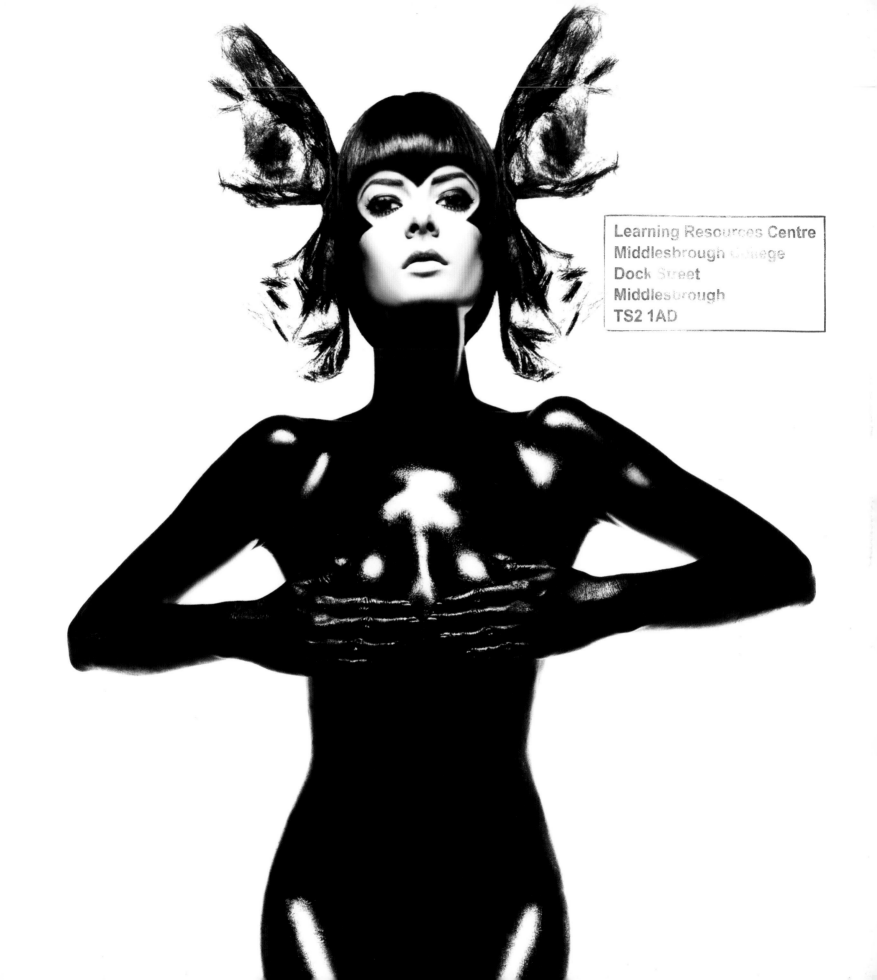

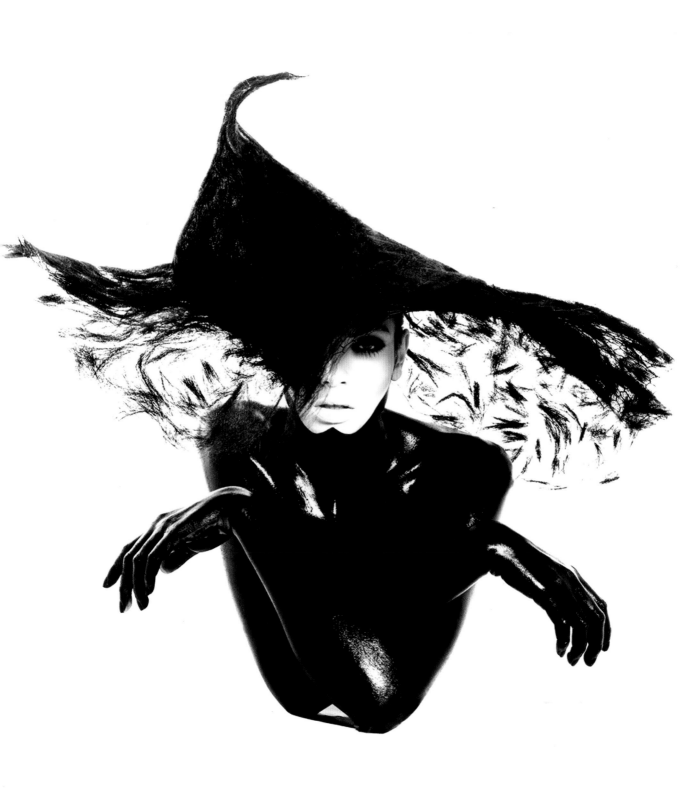

Creating the Look

For this shoot the models were to be dark and appear a bit like a silhouette, with light catching parts of the body. After considering black models, the makeup artist decided to achieve the look purely with cosmetics, first experimenting with different mediums.

1 For the face, Studio Fix Fluid by MAC, a matte medium-coverage foundation, was applied, with contouring done using MAC's Studio Sculpt; highlighting was achieved with Touche Éclat.

2 Black eyeliner was applied on the inside rim of the eyes, and a smoky eye created over the mobile lid into the socket using black gel eyeliner and matte black eyeshadow.

3 False lashes were applied on the upper and lower lashes and the eyebrows were drawn in black gel eyeliner.

4 Lips were blocked out, then highlighted using loose iridescent powder.

5 Next the model changed into a black G-string that could be thrown away afterwards and nipple covers to make her feel more comfortable. A disposable gown was on hand to keep the model warm. The body was prepped with Barrier Cream from Charles Fox.

6 Kryolan greasepaint in black was applied to the whole body using a sponge and smoothed with a large synthetic brush; the face was also outlined in greasepaint. The hands and feet were done last.

7 After the shoot the greasepaint was removed with a cream remover and baby oil; soap and water will only make the makeup more difficult to remove.

• Body hair on the model is undesirable, as the hair will show through the makeup. Ensure your model is hair-free in advance of a bodypainting shoot.

**Photography and
Hair:** Desmond Murray
Makeup: Jo Sugar
using Charles Fox
Model: Sophie Willing

UNDERWATER

There are many different scenarios where waterproof makeup may be required. You could be shooting on a beach, in a swimming pool or filming in a water tank on a film set. In most cases, the model will need to be retouched after just one shot in the water.

Working with water can be unpredictable and it is not always easy to guess how the skin is going to look or react when makeup and water meet, so be prepared to make changes. The key to successfully using and working with waterproof makeup is how you apply it and set it afterwards. It is important that all the skin on show is covered with foundation or a waterproof fake tan. Finish the skin with a specialist fixer spray and powder, which will help the makeup stay on longer in water. Sometimes a few blasts of hairspray can also do the trick.

Water reflects light and, depending on the type of shoot you are working on, the water can alter the colour of the skin, making it looked washed-out and colourless. This is especially true when working in deep water tanks. For best results and to combat this, use cream-based products and strong, vibrant colours to bring out the features. By mixing mediums with eye pigments it will give you a longer-lasting look, but these will tend to crack when worn all day.

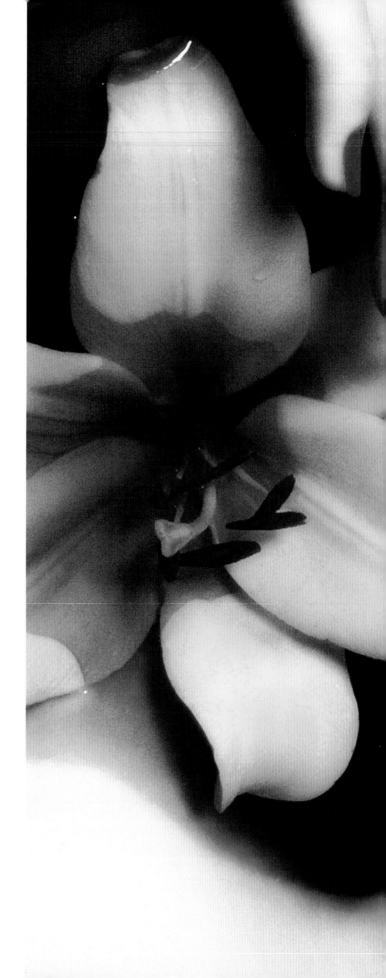

Photographer: Fabrice Lachant **Makeup:** Lan Nguyen using MAC
Model: Kate Willing
Makeup Assistants:
Kelly Mendiola and Karla B @ AOFM Agency

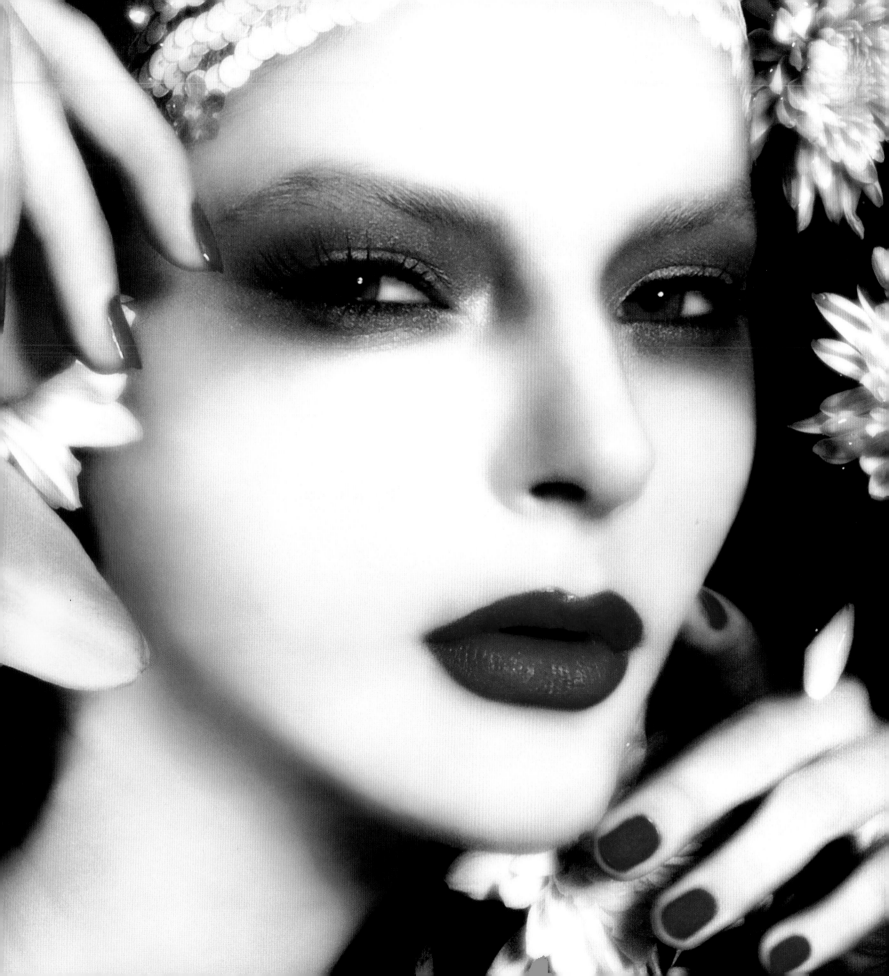

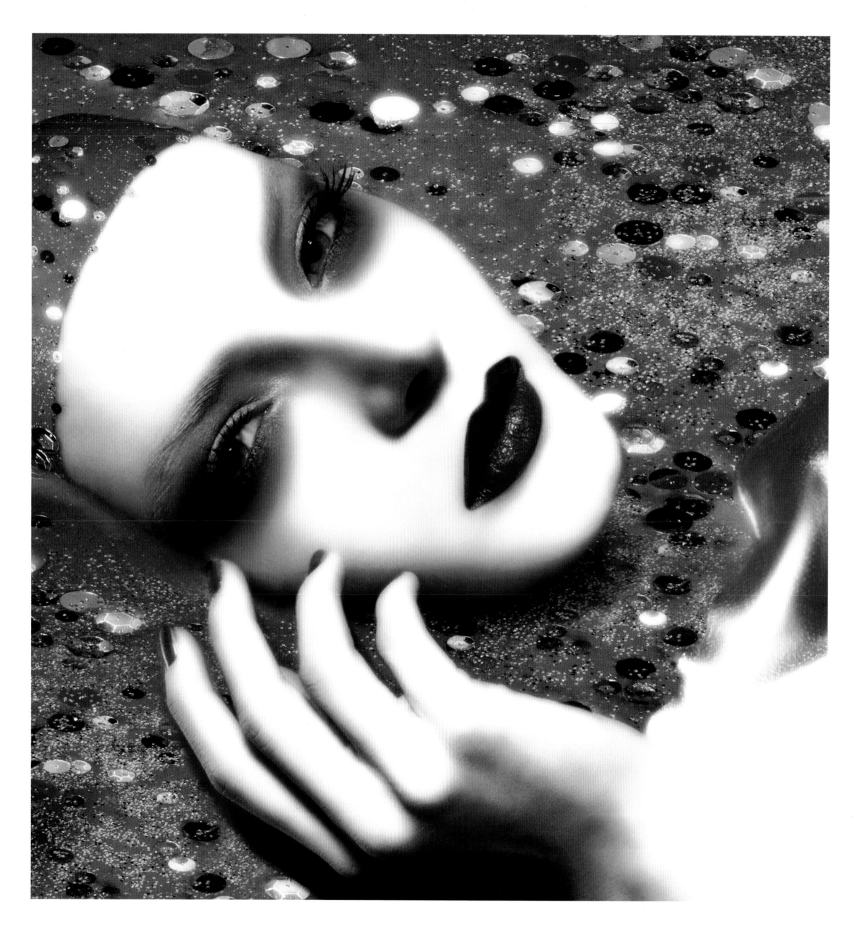

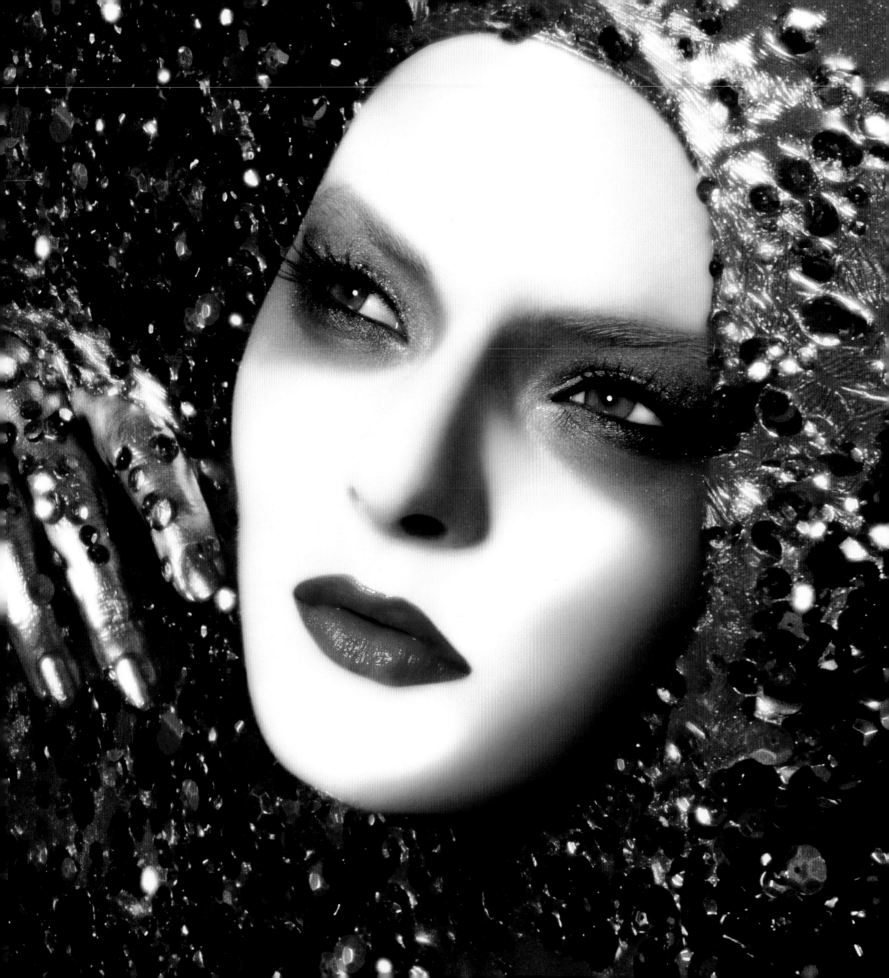

ADORNMENT

Makeup is evolving all the time and continues to be very experimental. By adorning the skin and using the technique of mixing paint and pigments you can create mask-like effects, which are visually inspiring. This can usually be seen in creative magazines and in jewellery advertisements where the face and piece of jewellery is the focus of the image.

There are alternative materials that can look interesting when applied to areas of the face, such as fabrics, beads, crystals, feathers and most art and craft materials. Crystals add a touch of glamour to a look, and when applied sparsely around the eye area can be wearable for a special occasion. For the best results, only use a small amount of glue, as too much will cause the stone to move and become messy. Duo adhesive glue can be used to stick these materials to the skin, as it is safe and easy to remove afterwards.

Photographer: Camille Sanson **Makeup:** Lan Nguyen using MAC and Swarovski **Model:** Ida @ Oxygen. Jewellery piece by Louis Mariette

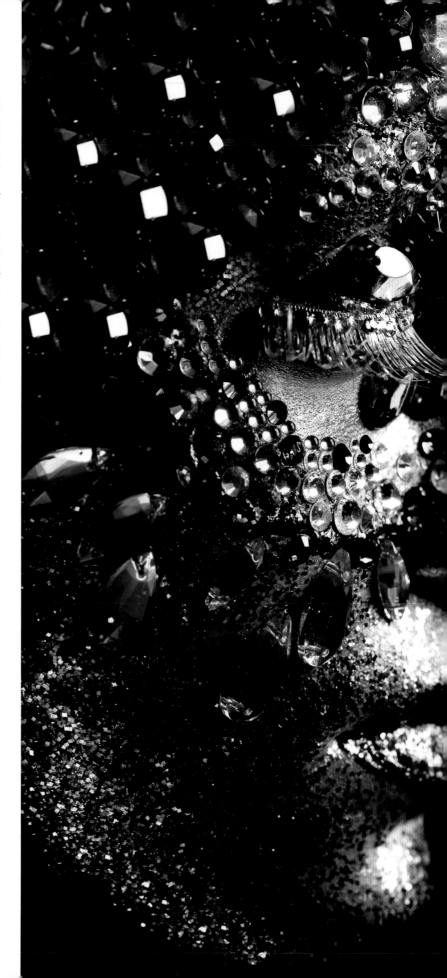

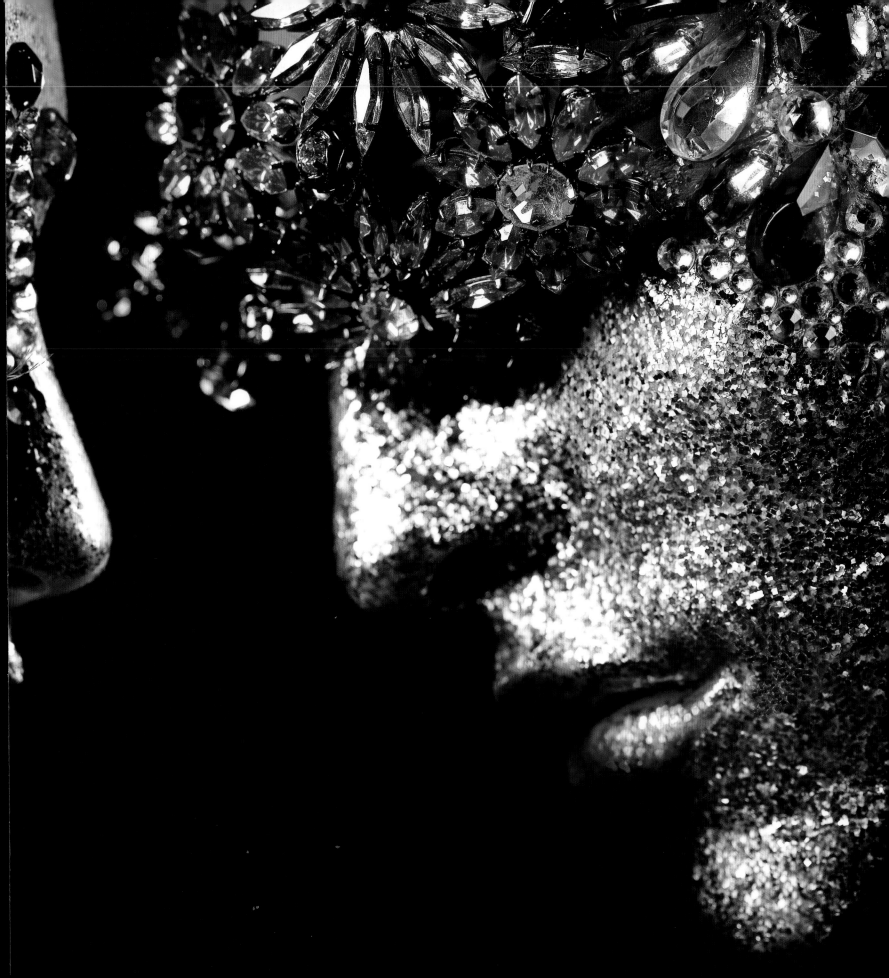

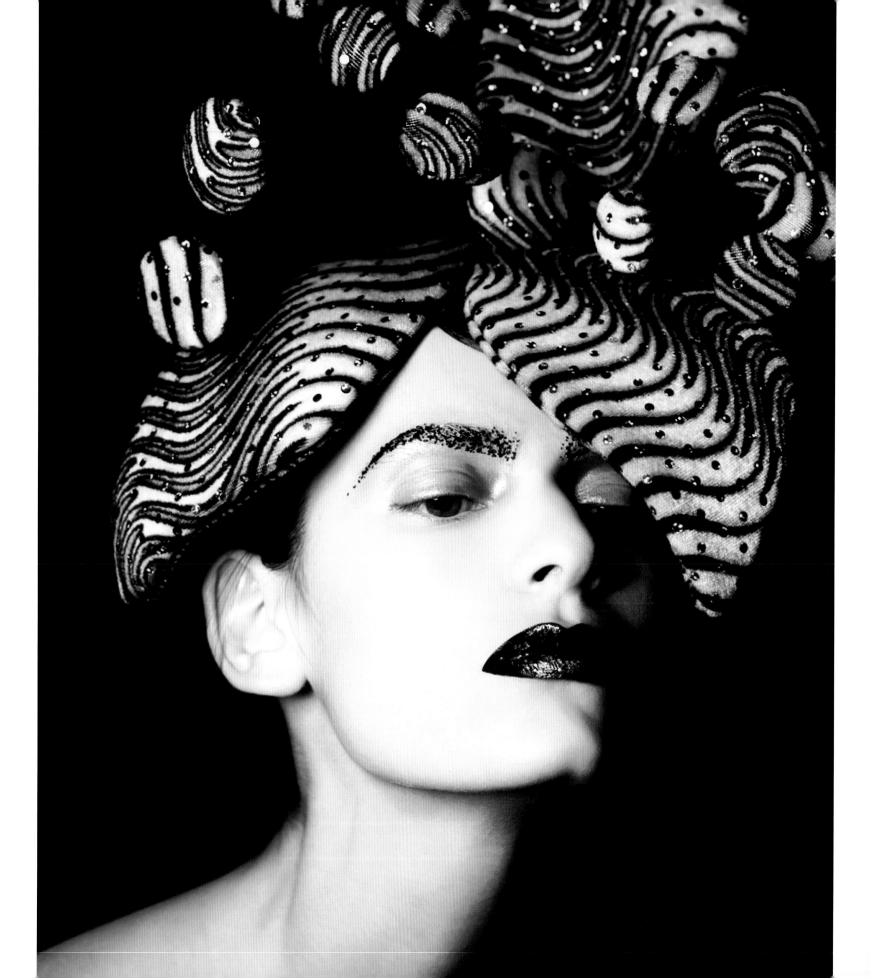

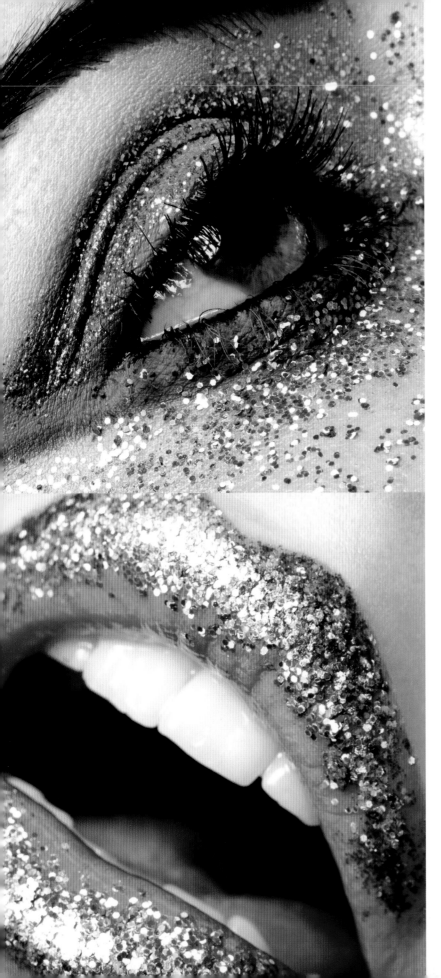

Working with glitter can often be a bit messy and tricky – loose glitter and pigments stick for a while, but will eventually fall off onto the face, depending on how much you use.

When you are using glitter around the eyes, use a cream-based eyeshadow, greasepaint or any product that has a wet consistency and place the glitter directly on top using your finger or a flat eyeshadow brush. You can use a mixing medium, such as a gel eyeliner, to stick glitter on small areas such as under the eyes. For larger areas around the eye, an option is to use a face-and-body mixing medium, which is easily spread and mixed in with the glitter to create a metallic effect. It stays wet a little longer so you can build the depth of glitter, layer by layer. To remove all traces of glitter use a water-based cleanser, such as Lancôme Bi-Facil instant cleanser or baby oil.

Natural Look

To achieve a natural shimmer and sparkle around the eye, dab the glitter onto the base lightly and put more on the inner eye for a brightening effect. Some fine shimmer glitters can be used on the cheekbones to create highlights.

Disco Look

For a party look like the one top left, make sure the base eyeshadow is strong and blended on top and underneath the eye. dab a little mixing medium on all over and quickly place the multi-tone glitter to set. You can control the intensity of the glitter by slowly adding more, bit by bit.

- Use masking tape to remove stray glitter from the face.

- Completing the eyes before applying the foundation will save time and avoid smearing.

(far left) **Photographer:** Camille Sanson
Makeup: Lan Nguyen using MAC **Model:** Olga @ Profile. Hat by Louis Mariette

(left top and bottom) **Photographer:** Catherine Harbour
Makeup: Lan Nguyen using MAC **Model:** Gabriele D @ Premier

USING GLITTER

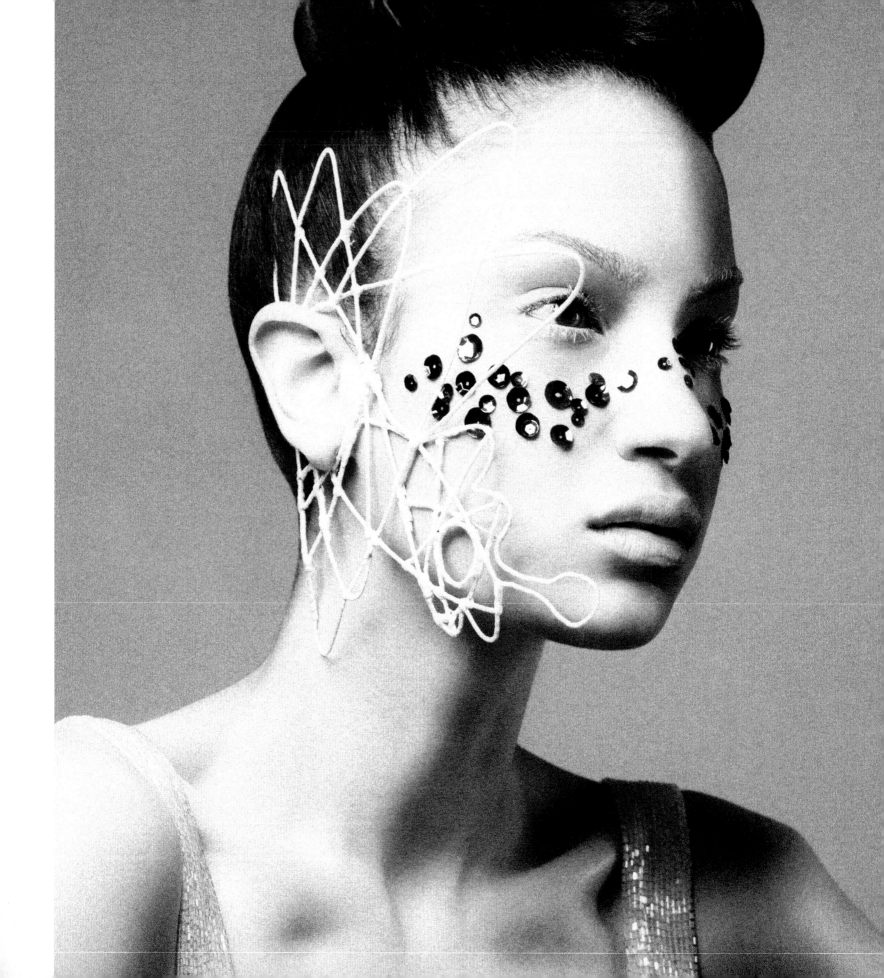

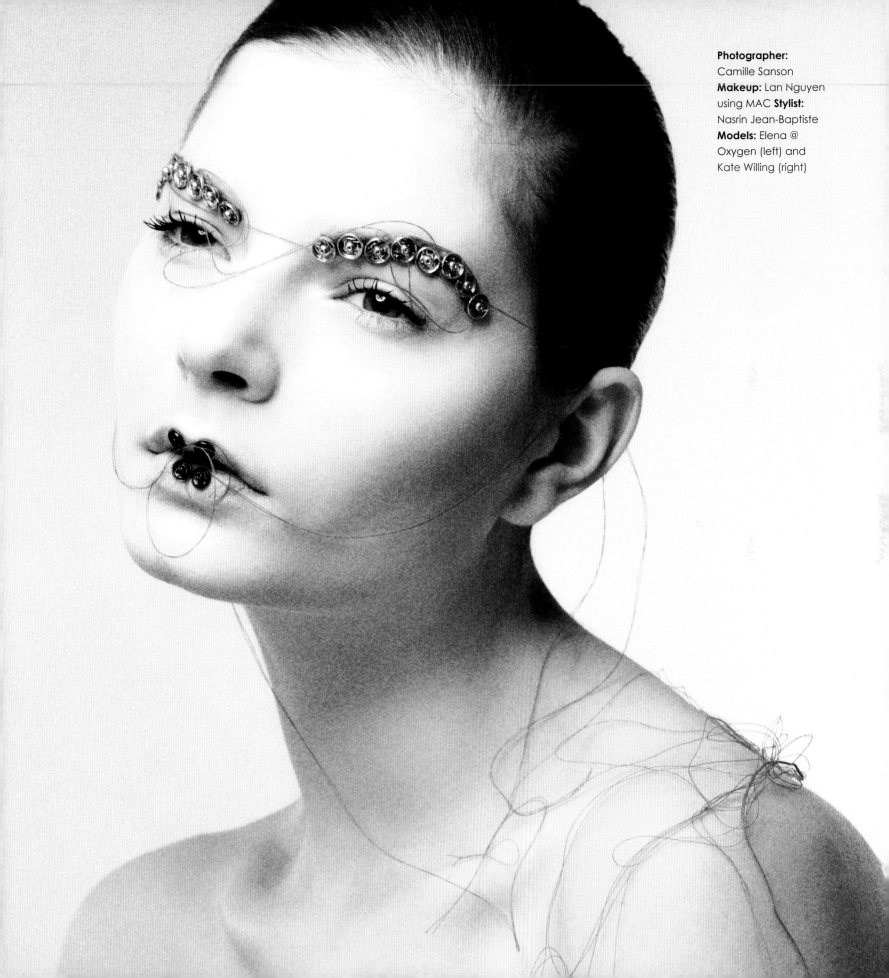

Photographer:
Camille Sanson
Makeup: Lan Nguyen
using MAC **Stylist:**
Nasrin Jean-Baptiste
Models: Elena @
Oxygen (left) and
Kate Willing (right)

WORKING WITH DIAMANTÉS

Using diamantés to adorn the face calls for plenty of patience. Picking each individual diamanté and placing it can be a long process – the trick is to use good tweezers. Choose flat-backed diamantés, otherwise they will not stick to the skin.

To save time, make sure you have a good idea of your design before you begin. The diamantés should be the last product to be applied once you have finished creating the rest of the look. Sketch out where you plan to place the stones; this is particularly important if you are using different colours and sizes of diamanté. For example, a big gem on the eyelid may not be a good idea as it can restrict eye movement and make the eye look sleepy. When working with coloured diamantés it is best to use a base colour makeup similar to the gems to give the look a solid finish, as the gaps between the stones can be visible and sometimes look untidy. If you want to achieve contrast though, then you need not worry about this.

Applying Diamantés

Use a transparent glue that dries to a rubbery consistency, such as Duo, which makes it easier to rectify mistakes and pull off badly placed diamantés. Alcohol-based glue takes longer to dry and can irritate the skin. Place a dab of glue on a tray or the back of your hand and use the tweezers to pick up a diamanté; dip the flat side lightly into the glue. You only need a dot, as too much glue can be messy and the diamanté will slide around, making it hard to position accurately. Once you have placed the first diamanté, continue positioning them side-by-side, ensuring that they are in line and evenly dispersed. Continue in this way until you have finished.

(overleaf left) Dress by Richard Sorger, leather floral head piece from Erickson Beamon, Swarovski leather choker from Renush

(overleaf right) Head piece by Louis Mariette, jacket by Louis de Gama, necklace by Raris, necklace by Swarovski Crystallized, necklace (worn on hands) from Erickson Beamon, selection of rings from Erickson Beamon and Swarovski Crystallized

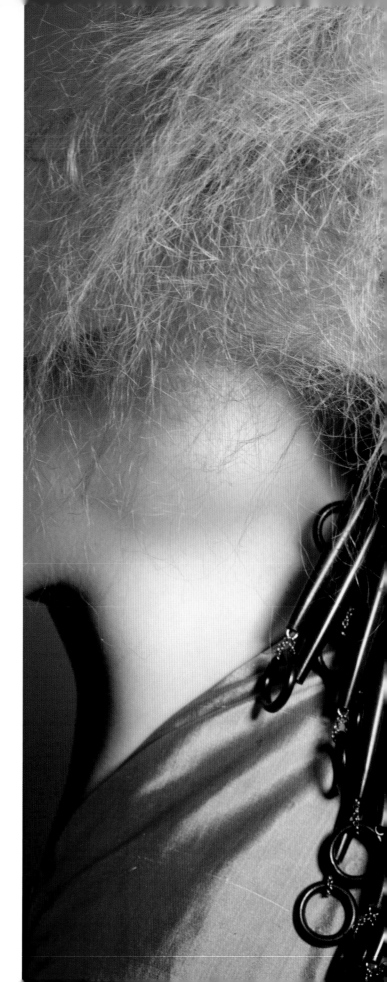

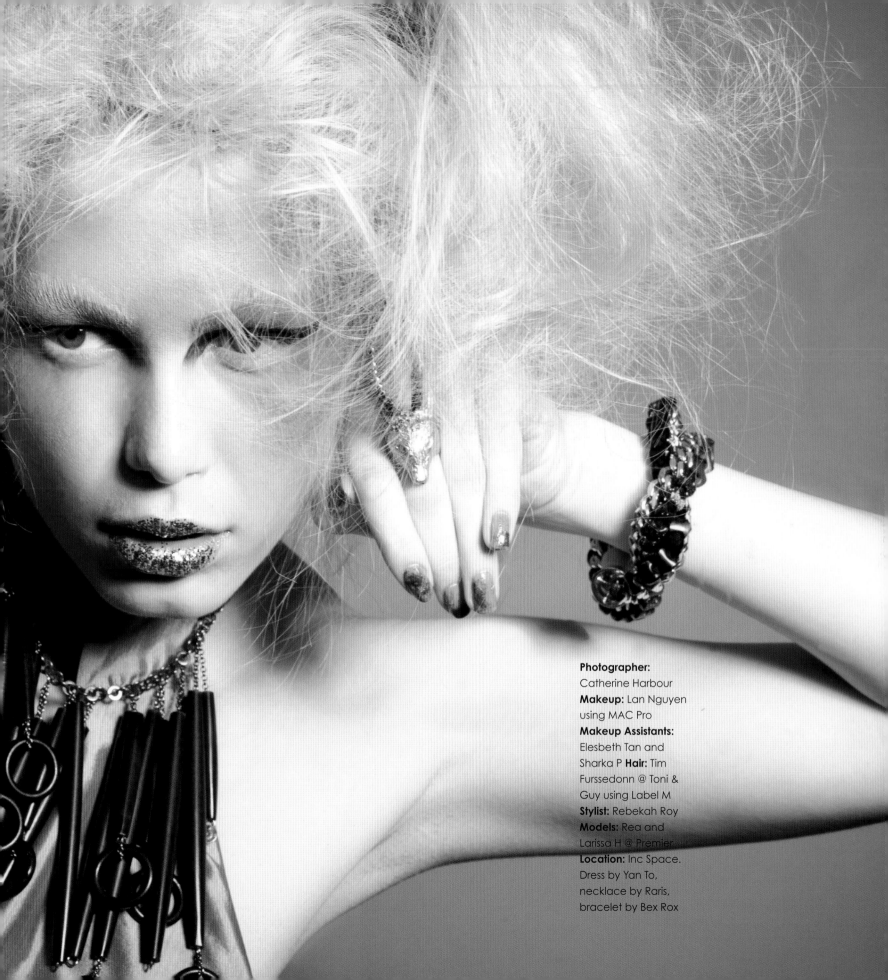

Photographer:
Catherine Harbour
Makeup: Lan Nguyen
using MAC Pro
Makeup Assistants:
Elesbeth Tan and
Sharka P **Hair:** Tim
Furssedonn @ Toni &
Guy using Label M
Stylist: Rebekah Roy
Models: Rea and
Larissa H @ Premier
Location: Inc Space.
Dress by Yan To,
necklace by Raris,
bracelet by Bex Rox

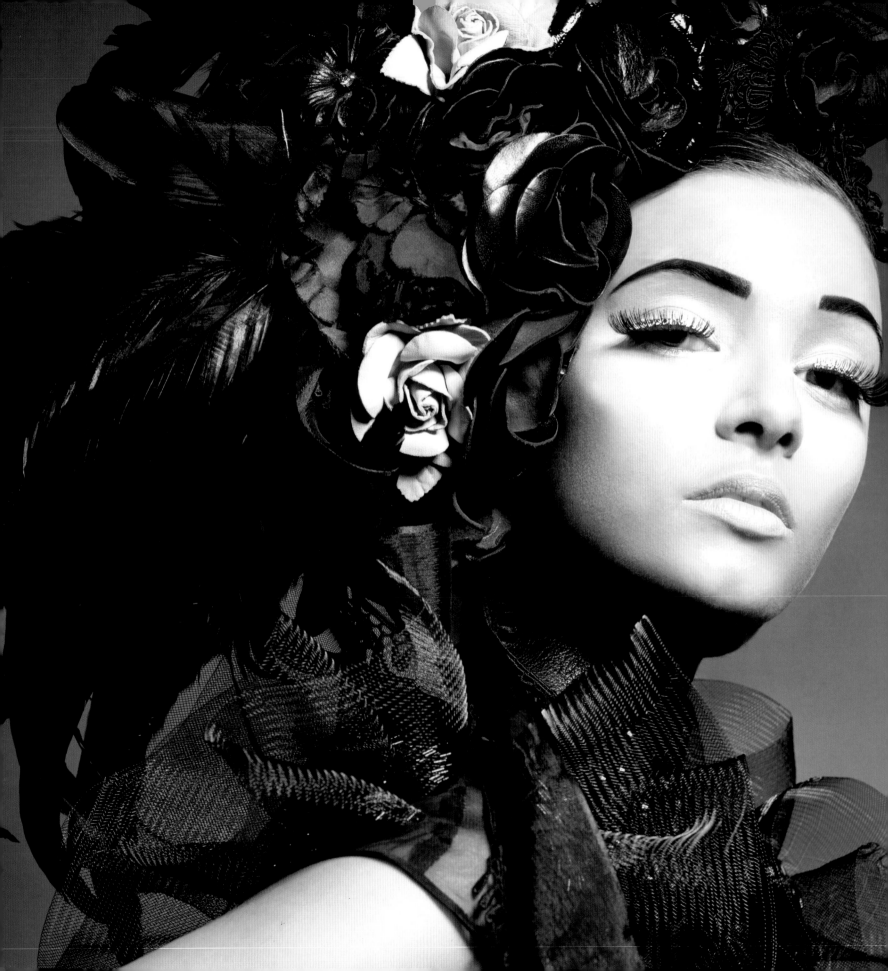

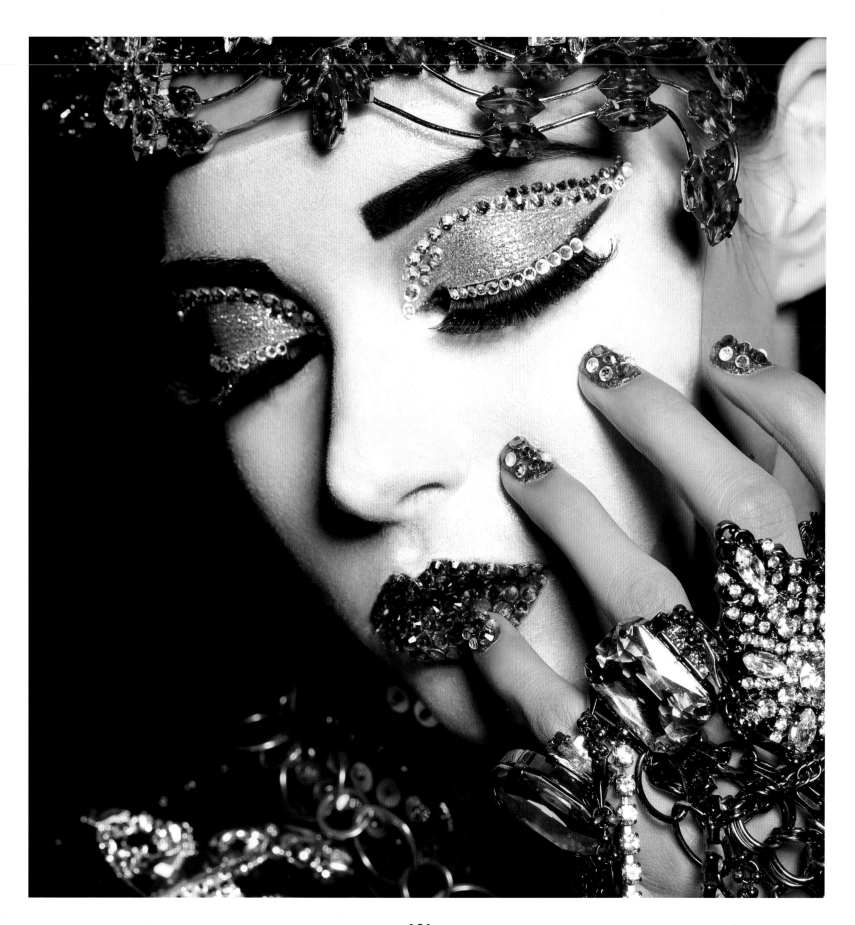

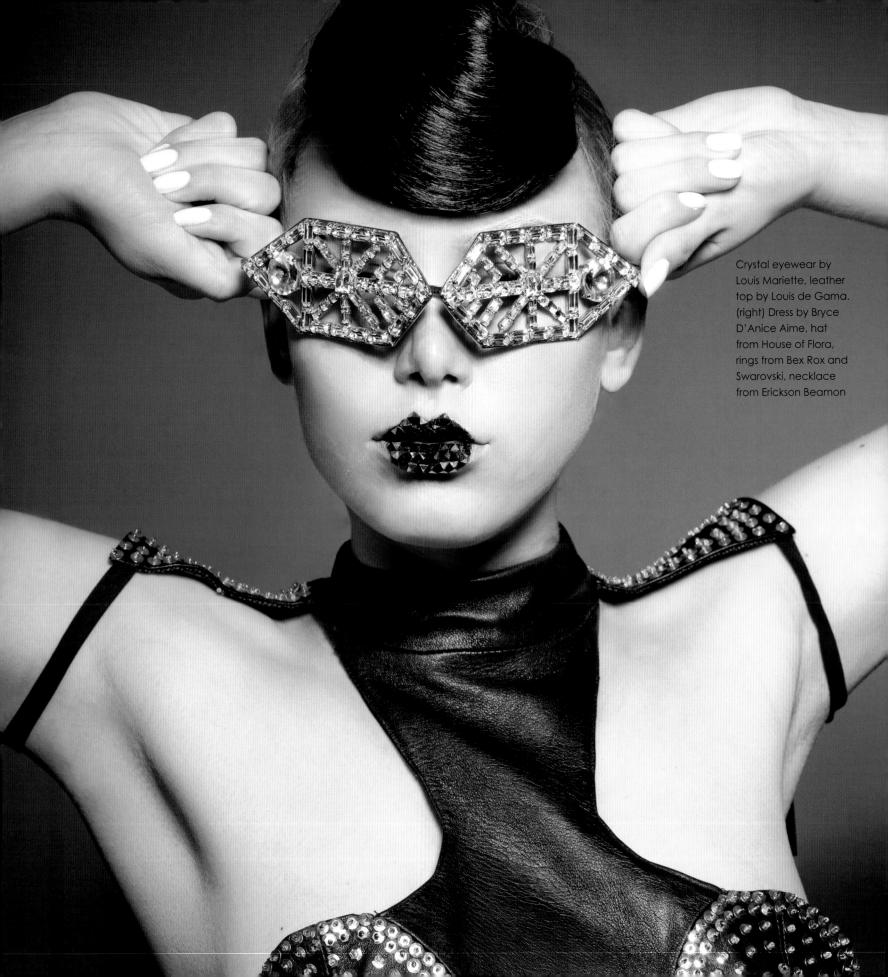

Crystal eyewear by Louis Mariette, leather top by Louis de Gama. (right) Dress by Bryce D'Anice Aime, hat from House of Flora, rings from Bex Rox and Swarovski, necklace from Erickson Beamon

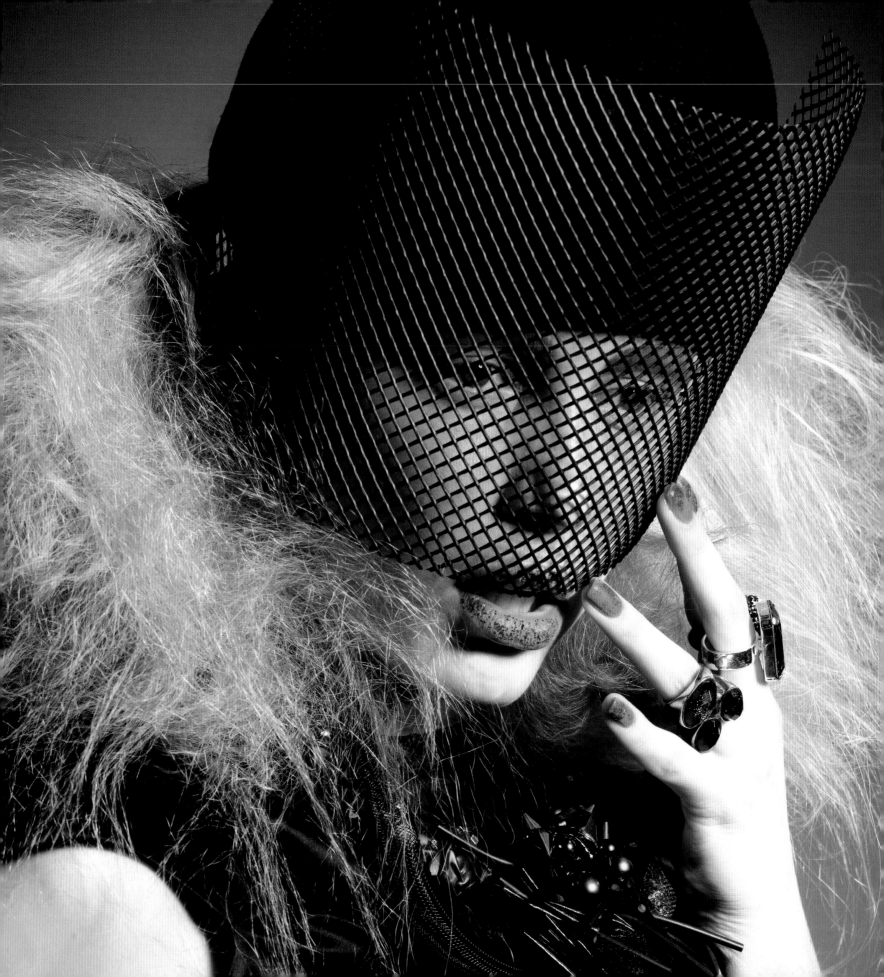

TOOLS

A makeup artist's kit is not just made up of makeup, but also includes a large selection of tools. These are essential to make the job easier and allow for the correct application of makeup.

Eyelash Curlers
An essential item in a makeup artist's kit, an eyelash curler needs to be used before mascara and, for maximum impact, used as close to the eyelid as possible (without pinching the skin). Heated versions are also available and can be used to curl stubborn, straight lashes. It is possible to heat metal eyelash curlers using a hairdryer, but these need to be tested for temperature on the inner forearm prior to applying to the eye. The most popular brand of eyelash curler is by Shu Uemura, which also manufactures mini eyelash curlers, great for curling the odd, stubborn, straight lash.

Tweezers
Besides tidying up eyebrows, tweezers are needed for applying false lashes and working with latex glue, such as Duo eyelash adhesive. Makeup artists will also use tweezers and Duo for applying intricate crystal-, bead- and feather work to the face.

Masking Tape
Handy to remove glitter fallout that may be stuck to the face or clothes, masking tape can also be used to create precise straight lines or graphic shapes on the face.

Bags
The most efficient way to transport all the materials a professional makeup artist needs for a job is in a suitcase on wheels. Not only does it hold all the kit you need (and spares),

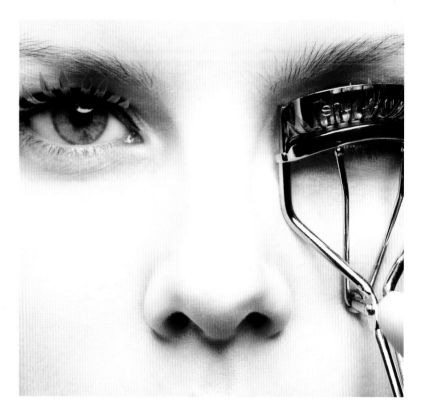

but it is a far easier and safer way to carry the heavy load. Most makeup artists will organize their kit into clear makeup bags, with similar products grouped together, to be able to see what products are available and to know where to find the products easily and quickly.

Other Essentials
For a full kit, you will also need disposable items, such a tissues, cotton buds, cotton pads, baby wipes (handy for cleaning hands and kit), and basic face wipes for when makeup needs to be removed quickly.

Photographer:
Camille Sanson
Makeup: Lan Nguyen
using Shu Uemura
Model: Erin @ Nevs

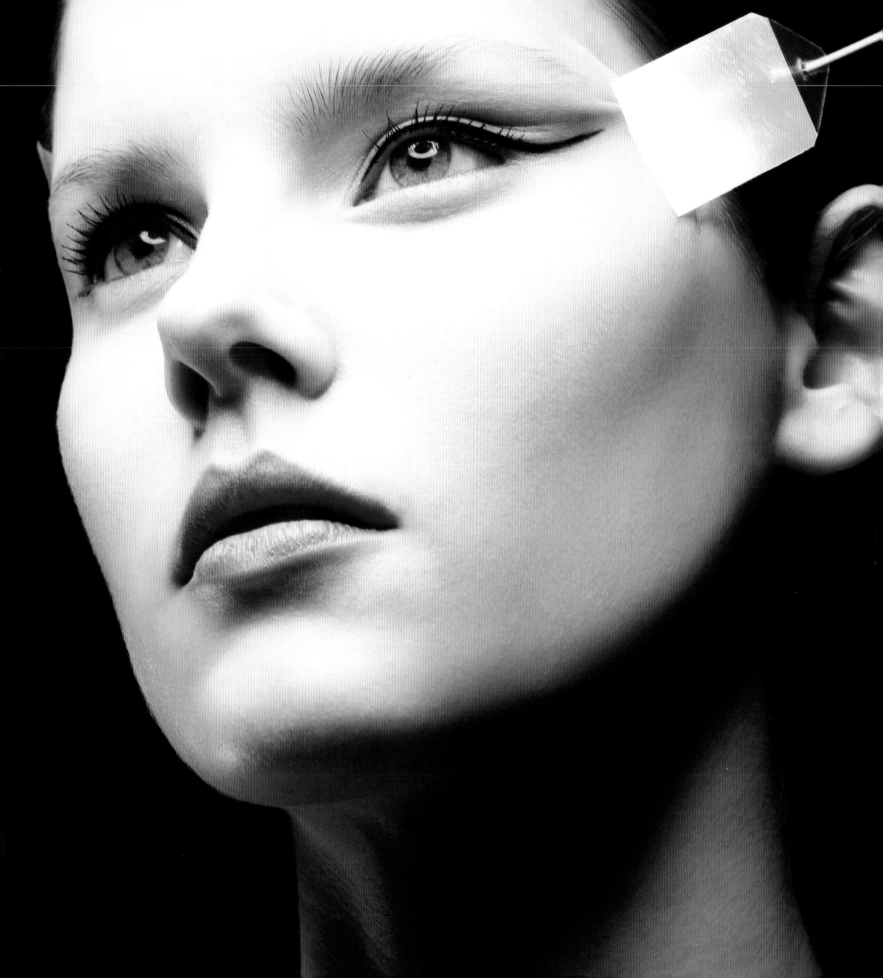

MAKEUP BRUSHES

Brushes are probably the most important tools in a makeup artist's kit. Not only do they help apply makeup with accuracy and precision, but they also allow the artist to blend and move the product to create the desired effect. Brushes come in a variety of different hair types, as well as sizes and shapes for various application use. The product formula determines which brush is suitable for use. Most makeup artists will have a large selection, and sometimes several of the same of their favourite brushes.

Cleaning Brushes

Cleaning brushes between applications is essential, both to remove product and to sanitize the brushes. A good, simple, alcohol-based brush cleaner, such as isopropyl alcohol, will kill bacteria instantly and dries in seconds, making the brushes ready to reuse.

All brushes AOFM Pro Tool.

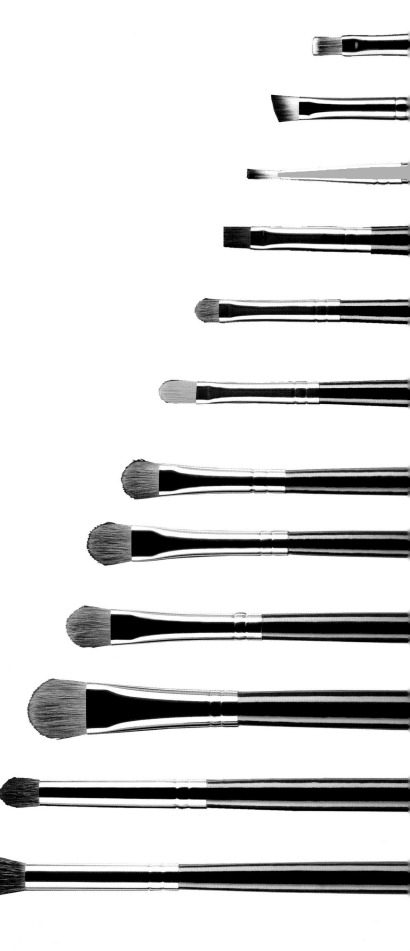

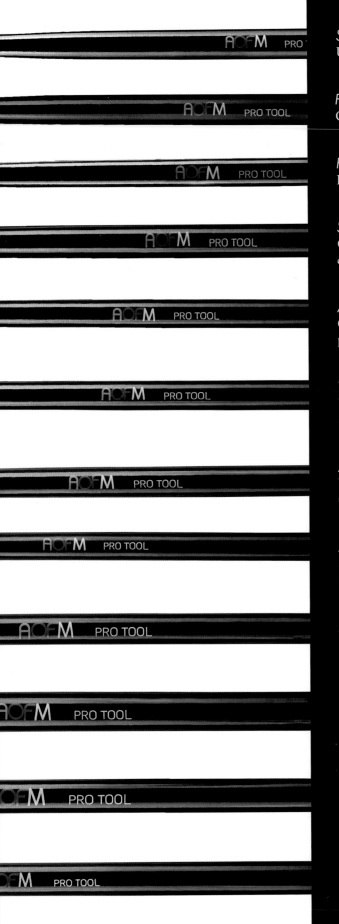

SMALL CONCEALER BRUSH (synthetic)
Used to apply spot concealer or liquid liner.

FINE BROW BRUSH (synthetic)
Creates sharp or natural-shaped eyebrows.

FINE LINE BRUSH (synthetic)
For liquid or gel eyeliner.

SPOT CONCEAL BRUSH (synthetic)
Can be used for lipstick application or to apply
concealer to a blemish or a specific area.

APPLICATION BRUSH 5 (natural)
Can be used to apply eyeshadow into small areas or
put shimmers or shadows into the corner of the eyes.

THREE-IN-ONE BRUSH (synthetic)
Useful for concealing spots and applying liquid eyeliner
and lipstick.

APPLICATION BRUSH 4 (natural)
Used to apply powders and eyeshadows with precision.
Can be used to apply a strong eyeshadow colour.

APPLICATION BRUSH 3 (natural)
Slightly wider application brush that can be used to apply
a heavy colour all over the lid of the eye.

APPLICATION BRUSH 2 (natural)
Applies powders and shadows with precision. Can be
used to apply a strong eyeshadow colour.

APPLICATION BRUSH 1 (natural)
Wider application brush that can be used to apply
a heavy colour all over the lid of the eye.

ROUND TIP BRUSH (natural)
Blends eye pencils for a smoky effect and can also be used to blend
hard lines.

CREASE BRUSH (natural)
Creates soft, smoky eyes or softens hard lines. Blends eyeshadows.

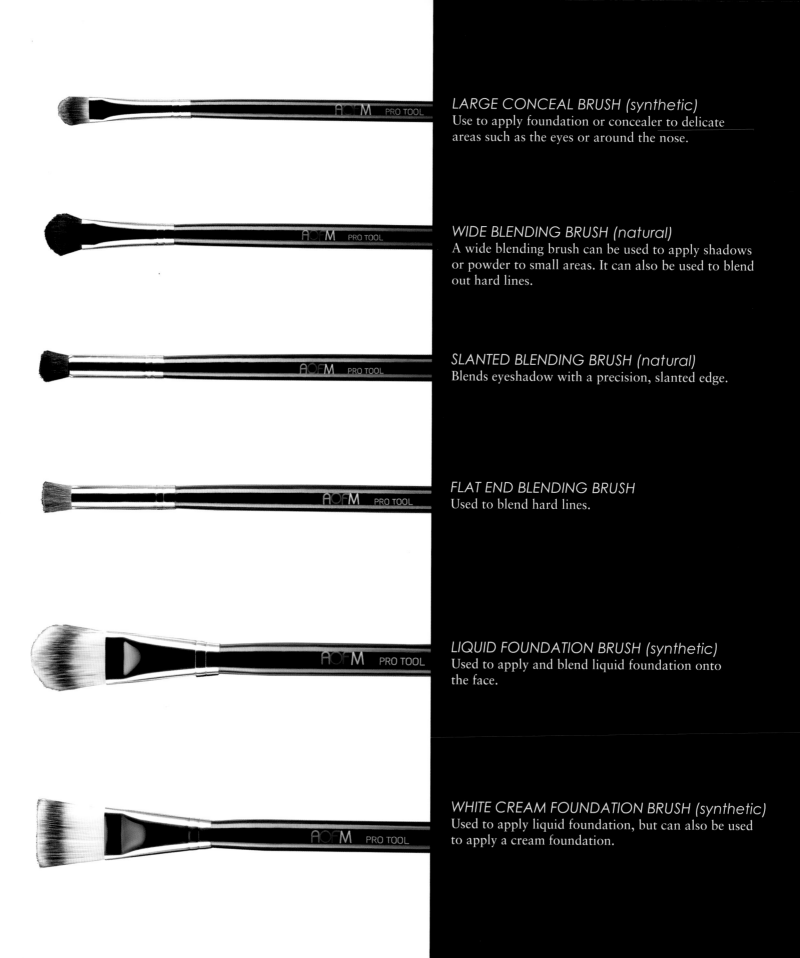

LARGE CONCEAL BRUSH (synthetic)
Use to apply foundation or concealer to delicate areas such as the eyes or around the nose.

WIDE BLENDING BRUSH (natural)
A wide blending brush can be used to apply shadows or powder to small areas. It can also be used to blend out hard lines.

SLANTED BLENDING BRUSH (natural)
Blends eyeshadow with a precision, slanted edge.

FLAT END BLENDING BRUSH
Used to blend hard lines.

LIQUID FOUNDATION BRUSH (synthetic)
Used to apply and blend liquid foundation onto the face.

WHITE CREAM FOUNDATION BRUSH (synthetic)
Used to apply liquid foundation, but can also be used to apply a cream foundation.

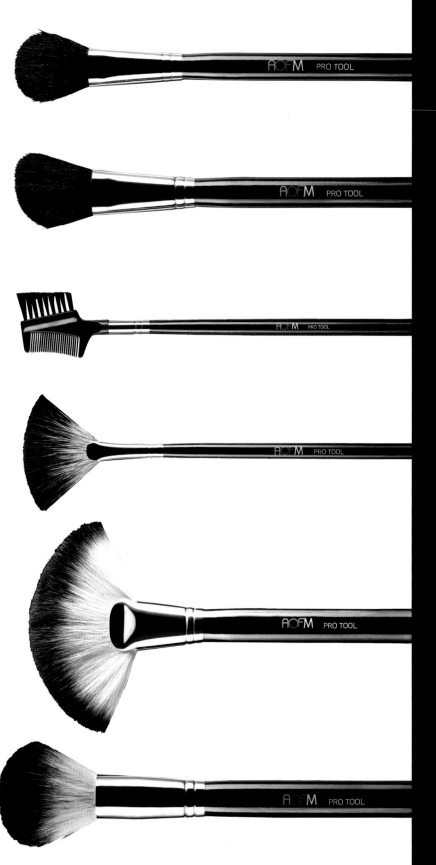

BRONZE AND SHADING BRUSH (natural)
For the application of bronzer, blusher or shading.

CONTOUR BRUSH (natural)
A slightly slanted brush to contour on the face, for bronzing, blushing or shading.

BROW COMB
Grooms and defines eyebrows.

FAN CONTOUR SHADING BRUSH (natural)
Used to sweep away loose pigment from under the eye, as well as to contour.

SIGNATURE FAN BRUSH (natural)
Used to apply loose powder to the face. Can be used to apply highlighter on cheekbones and can also be used to get rid of excess powder on the face or fallen eyeshadow.

BLACK AND WHITE POWDER BRUSH (natural)
For the application of loose or pressed powder.

What really happens before you see a runway show from either the front row, on the television or in the pages of a glossy magazine, can sometimes be taken for granted if you are not actually involved in the process. It takes dedication and months of hard work to prepare for such an event.

A long time before a model even sets foot on the catwalk there are meetings to discuss the trend forecasts, concepts and designs. Models, locations and crews have to be picked and tested and then the PR teams go into overdrive to make sure that key press teams come and cover the event. It is a cycle that has been going on for many seasons and one that will never change. As a makeup artist you cannot help but want to be a part of it all.

A makeup artist has an important role in the catwalk show, as it is their responsibility to make sure that the look complements the designer's collection without overpowering it and taking the attention away from the garments. The look needs to be beautiful and fresh, but it also should be as new and exciting as the clothes because these looks will be the guidelines for next season's trends. Beauty editors from across the world will be using snapshots of the catwalk shows as references in their editorial, and let's not forget the celebrities that are in the front row – if they see a look they like, then you never know what may happen.

The head makeup artist for the show will have spent weeks designing mood boards and collaborating with the chief designer, fashion stylist and hair stylist to come up with the various looks. Mood boards are a kind of collage of images that designers put together to create a visual guide and inspiration for their collection. Very often the designer and stylists will email them to the key makeup and hair styists to give an idea of the feel of the new collection of garments and what kind of atmosphere they want to create for the show. This in turn gives the makeup a guideline and basis on what they are going to design in a way of a makeup look for the show.

A "test" is where they will have a practise run on a model. The hair and makeup will try out their designs and tweak it on the model until everyone is happy with the final look. The designer will try an outfit or two on the model from the new collection to check that it all meshes well with the hair and the makeup and the stylist is there to ensure it's all put together well – they are the ones who often source the shoes, tights, jewellery, and so on. They also help in deciding which outfit goes best on each model for the show.

Also before the show, the designer and stylist hold a "casting", a kind of interview/audition where models are seen by the designer, asked to try on an outfit and walk for them to see how they would potentially move on a runway.

Products and Brands

Product sponsorship can play a major role in how a makeup artist designs the look for a show. A cosmetic brand could be the one who pays the makeup artist for using their product at the show and also supplies the makeup for the team backstage, so the artist has to ensure that the look is created with products from that particular cosmetic brands line. For example, if designer David Koma's show is sponsored by Benefit and he asked for red-coloured eyes, then it's up to the makeup designer to create this look using a Benefit product such as Benetint (which is a red-cheek stain). Often a cosmetic brand will arrange press interviews backstage during the show to ask the artist what brand products they used for the show.

In preparation for the show, the makeup artist will be in contact with their product sponsor and order the amount of products he or she will need for the show. This is usually estimated by how many models there are and how many makeup assistants the key artist will have. Every makeup artist works differently but the average is one makeup assistant for every two to three models.

Makeup assistants can be pulled in from the head makeup artist's agents or a brand such as MAC can offer a team to work backstage. Sometimes if a brand such as AOFM is sponsoring the show, they can provide makeup assistants for the artist. Most makeup artists will have a sort of "first" assistant. This is a makeup artist who works with them often. This artists knows the head artist's makeup style and what products they like to use best, as well as how their kit is set up. They can help run things for the head artist when it gets very busy backstage.

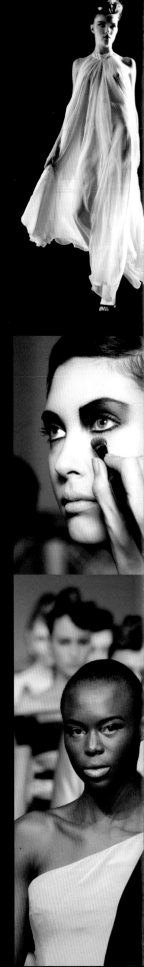

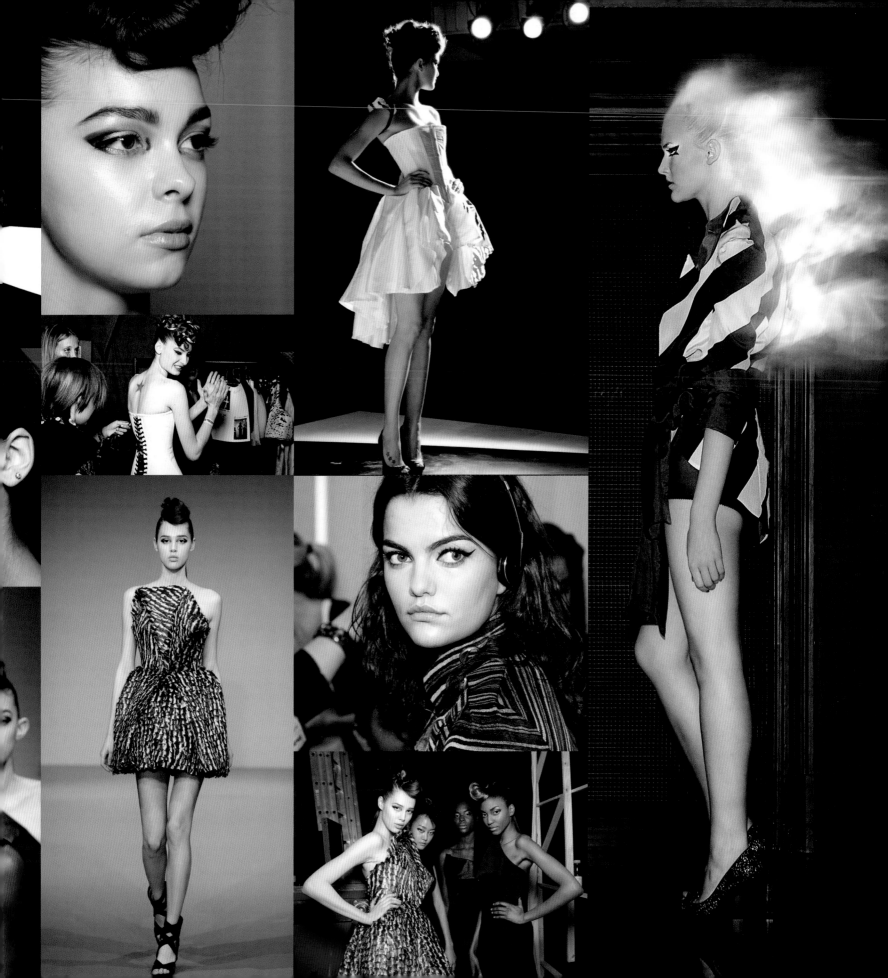

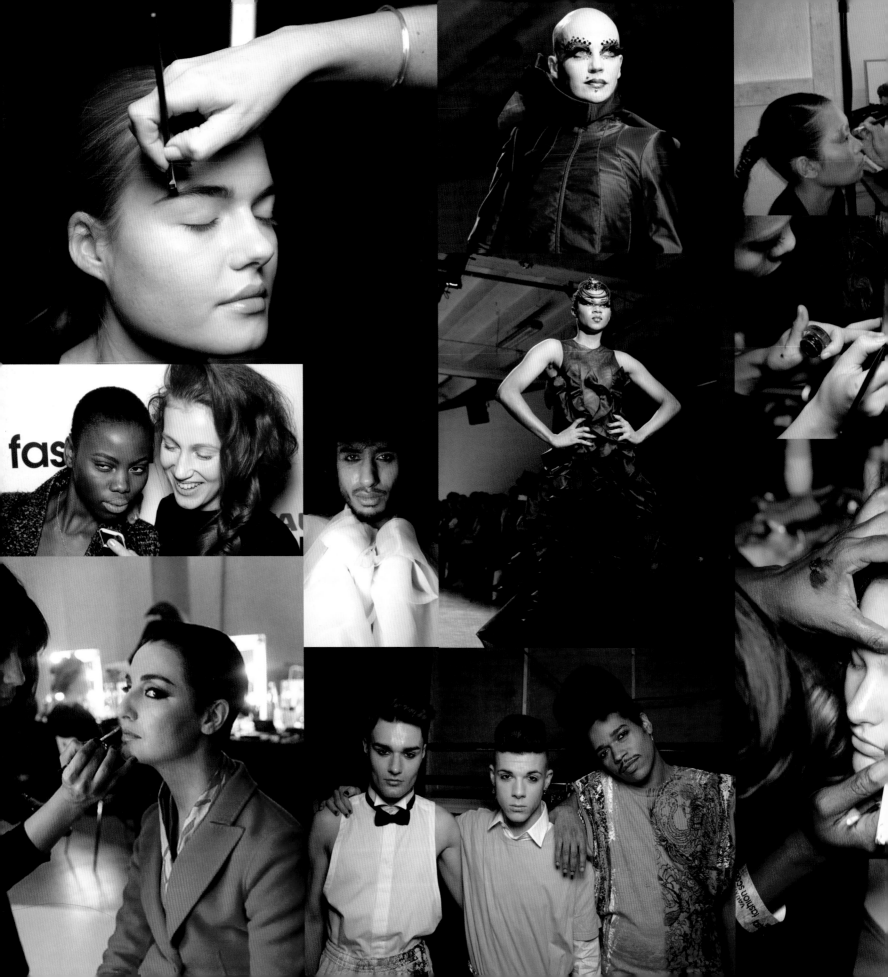

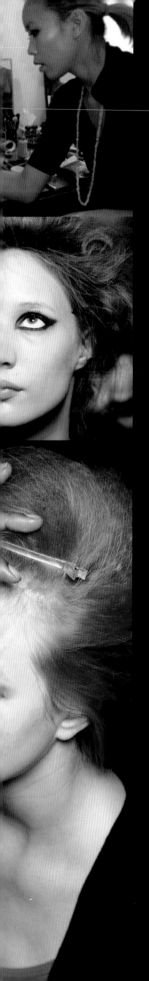

Both the head makeup artist and the makeup assistants are required to bring their makeup kits to ensure that they have everything they need to create the looks.

Four hours is the average time to prep before a fashion show and this is used for both the makeup and hair and last-minute clothing fittings on the models. At the start of the working day, the key makeup artist will use one of the models and do a "demo" on a model to demonstrate the look for the show. The head artist will show the key products to be used on all the models. It's imperative that the makeup assistants show up on time to watch this demo so they know what the look is for the show. They in turn will re-create this look on the models. Each model is then checked over by the head artist and any corrections or finishing touches of the look are done. It is important that the looks are finished on time and are on spec, as there is nothing worse than seeing mistakes on stage. Finally there is a makeup test and full dress rehearsal. with the fashion show producer for the models so they know exactly what to do for the show. The makeup head and a few assistants will check how the makeup is looking on the models on the runway, this helps see if there are any imperfections, blending or changes needed.

Just before the show, there are final checks. Often each assistant is given a small job such as powdering or lip touch-ups. This is often during the line up just before a show starts backstage – where all the models are queued in order and wearing their first outfits just as they are to step out onto the catwalk.

Finally, it is important to be focused when working on a catwalk show, as backstage can be very chaotic with television crews interviewing stylists and the designers, beauty editors wanting to get a preview, photographers getting close-ups of the makeup and models running in and out, getting their hair done and having clothes fittings. There will always be elements that you have not planned for, but you will have to deal with them in best way possible, such as a model arriving late or having bad skin. However, when the music starts, the lights dim and the first model walks down the runway, everyone will be looking at something that you have helped to create and you realize it has all been worth it.

ON THE DAY

One of the best things a new makeup artist can do to advance their career is to assist an established makeup artist. They can learn new creative ideas, innovative ways to use their brushes and see what products other makeup artists favour in their kits. Most importantly, they learn the proper etiquette for being backstage at a fashion show or what is really required from the makeup artist on a photo shoot.

Being a Good Makeup Assistant

Show up with clean brushes and a basic makeup kit. Most of the time, especially on fashion shows, the head makeup artist will provide or have the key products required to complete the look.

Do not be late and try to be early if possible; a makeup artist will usually need to be the first person on a job. It is important to be set up and ready to go when the models arrive. If the shoot is for a magazine cover with a celebrity, you do not want to keep the star waiting for you! If a makeup assistant is working on a fashion show, they must be there on time to learn the brief or the look for the job.

Listen to instructions from the head makeup artist, the most frustrating thing for the head makeup artist is for their assistant to go off and do their own thing. If a client has asked for a particular look on a job and the makeup artist does beautiful makeup, but it doesn't fulfil the brief, they can lose the job or never be hired again.

If you are standing around doing nothing, always ask the makeup artist what else can be done. Cleaning brushes, making a cup of tea and holding hair pins are all tedious jobs, but need to be done and are always much appreciated on set. Doing those extra little things will make you stand out from other less-helpful assistants.

If you are assisting, you are working on the head makeup artist's job and with their clients. Behaving with a mature and professional attitude is essential. You should not be giving the client your makeup card for future work; that is seen as trying to steal a client from the head makeup artist and is definitely frowned upon. A makeup assistant's behaviour is a reflection on the makeup artist themselves.

If you are booked to assist on a job and something comes up so you are unable to do it, always call the makeup artist as soon as possible. Do not text or send an email. Picking up the phone is the professional thing to do, better yet suggest a replacement if possible. Keeping a good network of other makeup artists is a great way to boost your own career – often makeup artists get double booked and having a good circle of contacts generates more work for everyone.

Most established makeup artists receive around three emails a week from new makeup artists or students enquiring about assisting. So never forget that assistants are easily replaced, but a great one is invaluable.

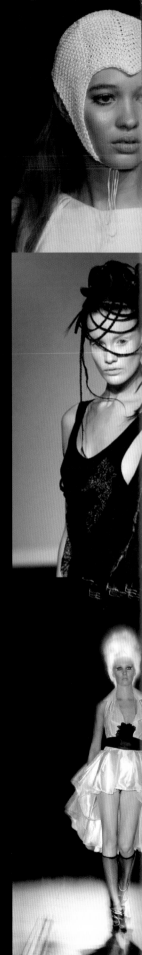

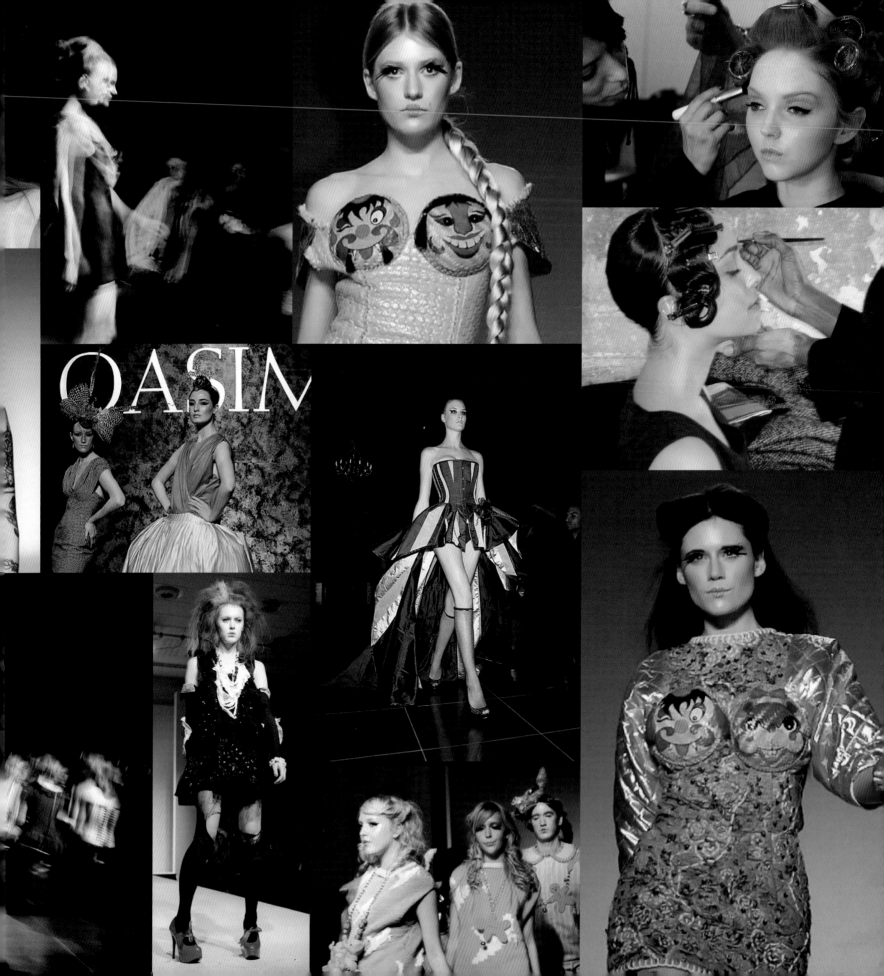

QASIM

QUESTIONS & ANSWERS

How do I become a successful makeup artist?

Training, assisting, testing and practising are all key to becoming successful, however being dedicated, having great contacts and continually networking are also essential elements to ensure you have a good chance of doing well as a makeup artist.

Do I need a qualification to work in the makeup industry?

In the UK, there is no standard form of accepted qualification in the freelance makeup industry. Many schools have their own form of certificate or offer NVQ, BABTAC and BTEC certificates. As there is no standard governing body, qualifications are not required by the industry to work as a professional makeup artist and they do not guarantee work. It really depends on the type of work you are pursuing.

If you are looking to join a makeup agency, work on a photo shoot with a new photographer or on a catwalk show, then you will be asked for your portfolio as proof of work and skills. Sometimes you will be asked to demonstrate your ideas or test the look before the actual shoot day. Your portfolio is really the only form of qualification accepted, especially within the fashion industry.

If you are seeking work with a makeup brand on a counter, companies prefer their sales staff to have some makeup training, but again it is not essential, as they would get the brand's makeup artist tutor to go through the techniques and concept of the looks that they want you to sell to the customer. Often there will be a few training days to show you the new products and trends for the season.

If you are working in the beauty, film and television industry in licensed premises, you may be asked to show both your qualifications and a CV/résumé. In film and television, a show reel will often be requested.

What does working freelance mean?

Working freelance is the same as being self-employed. It requires you to set up your own business and register your chosen name as a registered company. You pay your own salary and work directly with the client; you are in charge of paying your taxes and insurance. Being freelance, you have the freedom to do whatever job you like and work when you want to work. However, you have to be aware that you do not get the perks of being signed to a contract, where you would usually get holiday leave and sick pay.

If you do not work, you do not get paid, it is as simple as that. You always need to plan ahead for your next job so your diary is filled and you keep working. It is easy to get de-motivated and tiresome when you have to do all the paperwork and try and find work and also to be creative at the same time.

Being signed to a contract with a makeup agency offers you the security of having someone looking to help you grow and build your profile. They deal with the administrative side of your work, such as invoices and payments. They will also organize your diary and keep you in the heart of the industry, which is not easy since there are so many artists trying to do the same thing.

How does a new makeup artist get an agent?

Getting an agent can be very competitive. There are very few spaces per agency, but usually once a makeup artist lands one, it is far easier to get into another. A good way for a new makeup artist to get into an agency is to call them up and let them know they have just finished a makeup course and are available for assisting work. It is a good idea for you to have worked on a few tests first before approaching an agent, as they will probably ask to see your work. Very often, once a makeup artist is on an assistant list and they do well, there is room to move up into the agency in a shorter space of time.

How do I know where to get the best training possible?

If you are looking for a makeup school, there are several points to consider. The makeup industry is hard and very competitive; this cannot be stressed or highlighted enough. There are many schools claiming to promise you the world, however, it is up to you to create a successful career for yourself as a working makeup artist. No school can promise every student success.

Many academies claim to offer working makeup artists as tutors. Always ask to see the school tutor's current portfolios. If they cannot supply one, then it is doubtful they are current working fashion makeup artists. If they do supply one, then look at it closely – if they are not credited in a magazine or their work is not of magazine-quality, then they are not really top working makeup artists. It is no guarantee that schools with great pictures on their website use good makeup tutors who are active in the industry. Ask who will be teaching you and then do your own research on the tutor on the Internet.

Find out who supports the school – this can include big name cosmetic brands and hair companies. Any good school will be affiliated and will work with big name companies, as this shows they are highly regarded within the industry. If you are looking at schools claiming to offer international certificates that will ensure you will get work abroad afterward, be wary as there is no such thing as a fully qualified makeup artist, whether this is on a national or international basis.

A certificate alone will not guarantee work. There is no recognized international makeup association or qualification. The only association recognized by the leading UK schools is the National Association of Screen Makeup and Hair, (NADMAH, www.nasmah.co.uk.)

Schools are set up to act as a means of access to fast-track knowledge and an understanding of the industry – they do not qualify you to work. There are a number of top makeup artists in the industry, working on magazines like *Vogue* and television and feature films, with no previous makeup training, but who have become very successful.

Find out what cosmetic brands the school offers you to work with during your training. If a school only offers one make, you will be stuck in the industry, as no makeup artist will ever use just one brand. Your training should give you an understanding of all the products a professional would use. Be cautious of schools that offer kits, as in many cases they are not professional products and you can end up in a situation where you are not confident or comfortable using these products. Once you complete your training, you should have a good working knowledge of all beauty products.

It is important to see what past students have achieved from the school. Ask to meet current students, as this will give you a good insight into whether the school offers the right education for you. Student testimonials mean nothing and can be manipulated to sound better, so you must get all the facts right before you decide to part with your money.

Often on a course, you will be offered the chance to shoot your own portfolio to get you started, which will mean working with a model and photographer. It is important that you see the quality of images from past students, because this shoot will be the first chance you have to showcase your work. Can you visualize it in a magazine? Does the model look professional?

As a student, you will be paying a lot of money for your training, so you deserve to get the best teachers, products to work with and after care that money can buy. Many students assume that a career within the makeup industry comes straight after training. This is often not the case, as you still need to build up your practical experience.

Now I have trained, what is the best way to build a professional makeup kit?

Putting together a professional makeup kit when starting out can seem daunting and costly, but build it up slowly and it will not be as scary as you may think. When starting out, it is important not to buy the most expensive materials until you need them. It is advisable that students buy good-quality foundations, concealers and eyeshadows with good, strong pigment as a base first. As for lip glosses, lipsticks and other bits and pieces, it is better to go for a cheaper version to start with and invest in them as you get more experienced. When you start working with big-name designers, magazines and high-profile events, many press agents for cosmetic companies will give you products in return for a credit, which is also a form of advertising for the brand.

How does a new makeup artist build up their portfolio?

After training, new makeup artists work on tests. These are unpaid photo shoots organized between the photographer, stylist, makeup artist and sometimes a hairdresser. The aim of a test is to produce new photographs that showcase the work of all of those involved. On a test, model agencies often supply one of their new faces for the shoot to help build up their book. From there, it is up to the individual makeup artist to contact the modeling agencies, letting them know that they have just finished a makeup course and that they are available to show their work from the shoot. In turn, the agencies will often call new makeup artists to work on tests with their models.

There are also lots of great Internet sites with postings from photographers looking for makeup artists to collaborate with them on tests. New makeup artists can also post their work credits and portfolio pictures here. Remember, your portfolio is your tool in guaranteeing you future work, but it is just as important to have business cards to hand out while networking, as you never know who you might meet. A large volume of the work freelancers get are usually by chance meetings, word of mouth and through friends.

It is also good practice to have a website to showcase your work. The more people that know you exist, the more work you will get and a better profile you will build up.

How can I get to assist a makeup artist?

Usually, when you have finished your training, you will have been given experience to assist your tutors on jobs. Some schools have an after care service where they will direct you to the right places for contacts and makeup agencies. It is up to you to motivate yourself and offer your time and help to a current working makeup artist.

It is important to try and get work with as many different artists as possible, to gain tips from them. Every makeup artist has their own style and steps to create a look, even if the outcome is the same. There are so many different techniques and clever shortcuts that you can only learn through experience.

Does a makeup assistant get paid?

Many makeup assisting jobs are unpaid, but the experience you can gain from them is priceless. A makeup artist can learn and develop new skills and build up their speed and confidence. After assisting makeup artists for free, small paid jobs and clients are often passed on to the assistant.

How long will it take until a new makeup artist starts making money?

It is hard to say exactly, as each makeup artist's career varies. It really is a mixture of luck, determination and talent. Some makeup artists may already have industry contacts, while others will have to knock on a lot of doors to be given chances, but if you are willing to do the legwork it usually pays off.

The majority of makeup artists will say it took them two to three years to start getting some better-paid makeup jobs. Remember that during this time, a new makeup artist is testing for free and spending money building up their kit, so a part-time job in the industry would be a good idea to help fund this.

How can I ensure I get work in such a competitive industry?

It is best to focus on a certain area in the industry and excel in that. As a makeup artist you will get jobs in other areas, but when you are starting out, you need to realize where your skills are best suited within the industry. the retail industry, your personality and ability to understand the needs of a customer, who does not know much about makeup, plays a vital role. It is important to understand that you are working with all different types of skin and ages. Product knowledge of the brand is essential and you need to know how to sell the brand by recommending the right products for your customer. You will need to have a CV/résumé and an interview with the store manager, then if you are successful you will receive formal training. There are plenty of brands to work with, so choose one that you can see yourself working with and contact the manager directly.

In television, film and theatre, the work is regular and you get perks, such as a regular salary and benefits. These jobs are less widely available as they tend to be long-term contracts of at least six months. To get into this field, you need to send your CV/résumé to the head makeup designer and then offer to assist. In theatre, you would also be expected to groom wigs, cut hair and work with the wardrobe mistress. Offering your services and working in other fields, such as production, where you just help out and do what you can, will help establish you as a member of the team. You may just get a lucky break, too.

The fashion and catwalk industry is renowned as being very competitive. Your success depends on your own creativity, how much exposure your profile has had and your previous experience in working with big names. Do not be overwhelmed. It can be frightening, as your skills and portfolio are often judged before you have even had the chance to meet the client. The best way is to research makeup agencies and find a few artists that you aspire to be like, then offer your assistance. It really is who you know that can get you the big jobs because they are rarely advertised. A lot of artists get their work from being recommended by a photographer, stylist or a client they have worked with before. Networking at exclusive launches and parties are all vital parts of your work, as people like to put a face to a name.

Bridal makeup is done primarily for the camera and only secondly for the naked eye (the guests). The bride will continuously look back at the pictures for the rest of her life, so it is important that she looks perfect in them. A traditional church wedding will require a look with soft colours, often a mix of pastel pinks and peaches, while ethnic weddings often require more vibrant colours.

It is important to have a wedding trial approximately one month before the wedding to determine what the bride wants. Work with tear sheets as the general public often do not understand makeup. Tthese tear sheets with help the bride picture what is suitable for her. As always, you should know what the current trends are, be able to make celebrity references, know your period makeup and understand different cultures. Keep a written and visual record of what products you have used in the past, so that everything runs smoothly on the day.

You will either work with a hairdresser or be required to do the hair yourself, and you may also be asked to do nails. You may be asked to bring assistants with you, depending on how many people you are required to makeup, so do not forget to factor this into your fee. It is normal to expect a deposit as weddings are often booked up to a year in advance. Make sure you are paid for the wedding trial separately, in case your bride changes her mind and cancels the wedding (it does happen). Ensure you have allowed enough time for makeup application and that you have talked through your schedule with the rest of the team.

On the day of the wedding, arrive early, be calm and be organized in order to put your bride at ease. Remember this is one of the most important days of her life, so make it a special experience for her. Prepare a touch-up kit, either for yourself or for the bride to use, and be prepared for last-minute changes. You may be asked to do additional makeup on the day, or you may be required to change the makeup into an evening look for the reception.

When you are starting out, contacts and networking are really important. Ask your friends if you can do their wedding makeup and always carry business cards. If you do a good job, you will get most of your clients through referrals. You will often get referrals from the bride or meet people at the wedding who love the makeup and are getting married themselves, or have a friend who is. Advertising in local or bridal press can help and having a website can be a real advantage. Get yourself into an environment where you can meet clients easily, a make over studio or makeup counter work can put you in direct contact with potential clients.

SOURCES & SUPPLIERS

MAKEUP

Barry M
1 Bittacy Business Centre
Mill Hill East
London NW7 1BA
UK
Tel: 020 8346 7773
www.barrym.com

BECCA
Becca (London) Ltd
91A Pelham Street
London SW7 2NJ
UK
Tel: 020 7225 2501

Becca Inc.
132 Ninth Street
2nd Floor
San Francisco, CA 94103
USA
Tel: 415 553 8972

Becca Cosmetics Australia
Unit 4/36 O'Riordan Street
Alexandria
Sydney NSW 2015
Australia
Tel: (61) 2 8399 1274
www.beccacosmetics.com

Benefit
685 Market Street
7th Floor
San Francisco
CA 94105
USA
Tel: 1 800 781 2336 (phone orders)
www.benefitcosmetics.com

Greenwood House
91–99 New London Road
Chelmsford CM2 0PP
UK
Tel: 01245 347 138,
0800 496 1084 (phone orders)
www.benefitcosmetics.co.uk

Bobbi Brown
Estée Lauder
73 Grosvenor Street
London W1K 3BQ
UK
Tel: 0800 054 2988
(customer service)
www.bobbibrown.co.uk

The Estée Lauder Companies Inc.
767 Fifth Avenue
New York, NY 10153
USA
Tel: 1 877 310 9222
www.bobbibrowncosmetics.com

Chanel
Chanel Beauty Products
Rotherwick House
19–21 Old Bond Street
London W1S 4PX
UK
Tel: 020 7493 3836
www.chanel.com/en_GB

Chanel Inc.
15 East 57th Street
New York, NY 10022
USA
Tel: 1 800 550 0005
www.chanel.com

Charles Fox
22 Tavistock Street
Covent Garden
London WC2E 7PY
UK
Tel: 020 7240 3111
www.charlesfox.co.uk
see also Kryolan entry

Christian Dior
Marble Arch House
66–68 Seymour Street
London W1H 5AF
UK
Tel: 020 7563 6300
www.dior.com

Giorgio Armani
16, Place Vendôme
75001 Paris
France
www.giorgioarmanibeauty.com

UK
www.giorgioarmanibeauty.co.uk

USA
Tel: 1 877 276 2643 (customer
service)
www.giorgioarmanibeauty-usa.com

JESSICA
Gerrard International Limited
NNC House
47 Theobald Street
Borehamwood
Hertfordshire WD6 4RT

UK
Tel: 0845 2171360, 0845
2171360 (customer service)
www.jessica-nails.co.uk
www.jessicacosmetics.co.uk

Jessica Cosmetics International
12747 Saticoy Street
North Hollywood, CA 91605
USA
Tel: 818 759 1050, 1 800 582
4000 (customer service)
www.jessicacosmetics.com

Kryolan
Kryolan GmbH Papierstr.
10 D-13409
Berlin, Germany
Tel: (49) 30 499 892 0
www.kryolan.com

Kryolan Corp.
132 9th Street
San Francisco, CA 94103
USA
Tel: 1 800 KRYOLAN or
415 863 9684
www.usa.kryolan.com
*Available in the UK from
Charles Fox*

Lancôme
14 rue Royale
75008 Paris, France
www2.lancome.com/index.aspx

UK
www.lancome.co.uk

USA
www.lancome-usa.com

Laura Mercier
Gurwitch Products, LLC
13259 North Promenade Blvd
Stafford, TX 77477
USA
Tel: 1 888 637 2437
www.lauramercier.com

L'Oréal Ltd
255 Hammersmith Road
London W6 8AZ
UK
Tel: 020 8762 4000
www.loreal.co.uk

L'Oréal USA
575 Fifth Avenue
New York, NY 10017
Tel: 212 818 1500
www.lorealusa.com

L'Oréal International
41 Rue Martre
92217 Clichy Cedex
France
Tel: (33) 14756 7000
www.loreal.fr

MAC
73 Grosvenor Street
London W1K 3BQ
UK
Tel: 0870 034 6700,
0870 034 2676 (phone orders)
www.maccosmetics.co.uk

767 Fifth Avenue
New York, NY 10153
USA
Tel: 1 800 588 0070
www.maccosmetics.com

Make Up Forever
6 Goldhawk Mews
London W12 8PA
UK
Tel: 020 8740 6788
www.makeupforever.com

USA
www.makeupforeverusa.com
*Available at Sephora, see www.
sephora.com*

Nars
900 Third Avenue
New York, NY 10022
USA
Tel: 1 888 788 NARS
www.narscosmetics.com

UK
www.narscosmetics.co.uk

The Pro Makeup Shop
20 Mortlake High Street
London SW14 8JN
UK
Tel: 020 3178 2960
www.thepromakeupshop.com

Revlon
Greater London House
Hampstead Road
London NW1 7QX
Tel: 020 7391 7400

Revlon Inc.
237 Park Avenue
New York, NY 10017
USA
Tel: 212 527 4000
www.revlon.com

Screen Face
20 Powis Terrace
off Westbourne Park Road
London W11 1JH
UK
Tel: 020 7221 8289
www.screenface.com

Shu Uemura
55 Neal Street
Charing Cross
London WC2H 9PJ
UK
020 7836 5588
www.shuuemura.com

Yves Saint Laurent Beauty
34–36 Perrymount Road
Haywards Heath
West Sussex RH16 3DN
UK
Tel: 01444 255700
www.ysl.com

USA
www.yslbeautyus.com

MAKEUP ARTISTS

Carolyn Roper
www.getmadeup.com

Jo Sugar
www.josugar.com
Lan Nguyen
www.lan-makeup.com

Sandra Cooke
www.sandracooke.net/

Rachel Wood
www.rachelmakeup.co.uk

HAIR PRODUCTS

Bumble and Bumble
415 13th Street
New York, NY 10014
USA
Tel: 866 513 0498
www.bumbleandbumble.com

Babyliss Pro
The Conair Group Ltd
PO BOX 356
Fleet GU51 3ZQ
UK
Tel: 08705 133 191
www.babyliss.co.uk

USA
www.babylissus.com

KMS California
KPSS Inc.
981 Corporate Boulevard
Linthicum Heights MD 21090
USA
Tel: 410 850 7555,
1 800 342 5567 (phone orders)
www.kmscalifornia.com

KPSS UK Ltd
6 Park View
Alder Close
Eastbourne
East Sussex BN23 6QE
UK
Tel: 01323 413 200

KPSS Australia Pty Ltd
1A The Crescent
Kingsgrove NSW 2208
Australia
Tel: 612 9554 1900

Label M
Mascolo Group Ltd
Innovia House, Marish Wharf
St Mary's Road, Langley, Berkshire
SL3 6DA
UK
Tel: 0870 770 8080
www.labelm.co.uk

Redken
565 Fifth Avenue
New York, NY 10017
USA
www.redken.com

UK
www.redken.co.uk

TIGI
Tigi Australia Ltd
21/39 Herbert Street
St Leonards
NSW 2065
Australia
Tel: (61) 2 9439 9666
www.tigihaircare.com

Tigi Haircare Ltd
Tigi House, Bentinck Road
West Drayton UB7 7RQ
UK
Tel: 01895 458550

Tigi Linea
1655 Waters Ridge Drive
Lewisville, TX 75057-6013
USA
Tel: 469 528 4300

HAIR STYLISTS

Desmond Murray
http://desmondmurray.com

Fabio Vivan
http://fabiovivan.com/

Marc Eastlake
http://www.myspace.com/
thegentrysalon

Natasha Mygdal
http://www.natashamygdal.com

Zoe Irwin
http://head1st.net/zoe/

SKINCARE

Alpha-H
18 Millennium Circuit
Helensvale Q 4212
Gold Coast, Australia
www.alpha-h.com
Tel: (61) 7 5529 4866
www.alpha-h.com

Bio Oil
Union Swiss
66 Long Street
Cape Town 8001
South Africa
Tel: (27) 21 424 4230
www.bio-oil.com

Dermalogica
1535 Beachey Place
Carson, CA 90746
USA
Tel: 310 900 4000
www.dermalogica.com

Caxton House Randalls Way
Leatherhead
Surrey KT22 7TW
UK
Tel: 01372 363600
www.dermalogica.com/uk

111 Chandos Street
Crows Nest NSW 2065
Australia
Tel: 1 800 659 118 or
(61) 2 8437 9600

Kiehl's
54 Columbus Avenue
New York, NY 10023
USA
Tel: 1 800 543 4572 or
732 951 4545
www.kiehls.com

186A King's Road
London SW3 5XP
UK
Tel: 020 7751 5950
www.kiehls.co.uk

Rodial
The Plaza
535 Kings Road
London SW10 0SZ
UK
Tel: 020 7351 1720
www.rodial.co.uk

St Tropez
Beauty Source Limited Unit
4C Tissington Close
Chilwell NG9 6QG
UK
Tel: 0115 983 6363
www.st-tropez.com

PO Box 800876
Santa Clarita, CA 91380
USA
Tel: 1 800 366 6383
www.st-tropez.com

PO Box 334
Terrey Hills NSW 2084
Australia
Tel: 1 800 358 999
www.sttropeztan.com.au

Simple
Simple Health and Beauty Ltd
4th Floor Chadwick House
Blenheim Court
Solihull B91 2AA
UK
Tel: 0121 712 6523
www.simple.co.uk

FASHION & ACCESSORIES

Erickson Beamon
www.ericksonbeamon.com

Louis Mariette
http://www.louismariette.com/

Swarovski
http://www.swarovski.com

PHOTOGRAPHERS

Atton Conrad
www.attonconrad.com

Camille Sanson
www.camillesanson.com

Catherine Harbour
http://www.catherineharbour.com/

Dez Mighty
www.dezmighty.com

Fabrice Lachant
http://www.photobyfabrice.com

Han Lee De Boer
http://hanleedeboer.com/

Jason Ell
http://www.jasonell.com/

Keith Clouston
http://www.keithclouston.com

Lou Denim
http://www.loudenim.com

Roberto Aguilar
www.photoaguilar.com

Zoe Barling
http://www.zoebarling.com/

STYLISTS

Karl Willett
http://www.ilovemystylist.com/

Narin Jean-Baptiste
http://www.nasrinjeanbaptiste.com/

Rebekah Roy
http://www.fashion-stylist.net/

Samson Soboye
http://www.samson-soboye.com/

Shyla Hassan
http://www.shylahassan.com/

Svetlana Prodanic
http://svetlanastyling.com/

SPACES and SERVICES

Balcony Jump Management
www.balconyjump.co.uk

Blow PR
www.blow.co.uk

Disciple Productions
http://www.disciple-productions.
com

Escala Music
http://www.escalamusic.com/gb/

First Model Management
www.firstmodelmanagement.
co.uk

FM Agency
www.fmmodelagency.com

IMG Models
www.imgmodels.com

I.N.C. Space
www.inc-space.com

International Collective www.
internationalcollective.co.uk

M&P Models
www.mandpmodels.com

Modus Dowal Walker PR
www.moduspublicity.com

Nevs Model Agency
www.nevsmodels.co.uk

Next Models
www.nextmodels.com

No. 5 Cavendish Square
http://www.no5ltd.com/

Oceanfall Talent Agency
http://www.oceanfall.co.uk

Octagon
http://www.octagon-uk.com

Purple PR
www.purplepr.com

Salon Sensations
www.salonsensations.co.uk

PRODUCTS USED
FOR THE LOOKS

SKINCARE

Instant Results
Alpha-H White Gold Skin Brightening
Solution
Alpha-H Liquid Gold
Alpha-H Phase Three Clearing Gel
Elizabeth Eight-Hour Cream
Shu Uemura Deapsea Hydrability
Moisturizing Lip Balm

Exfoliators
Neutrogena Deep Clean Foaming
  Scrub
Clarins Gentle Exfoliator Brightening
  Toner
Dermalogica Daily Microfoliant
Alpha-H Micro Cleanse Exfoliant
Origins Modern Friction Face Scrub

Cleansers
Shu Uemura Balancing Cleansing Oil
Lancôme Gel Eclat
Chanel Gel Pureté Anti Pollution
Rinse Off Foaming Cleanser

Face Masks
Dermalogica Skin Hydrating Masque
Kiss My Face Organics Pore Shrink

Deep Pore Cleansing Mask
Clean & Clear Morning Burst Shine
Control Facial Scrub with Bursting
  Beads
Chanel Precision Masque Destressant
Purete Purifying Cream Mask
Lancôme Hydra-Intense Masque
Alpha-H 15% Glycolic Hydrating
Mask with Lavender

Pore Strips
Biore Pore Cleansing Strips.
Tea Tree and Witch Hazel Nose
  Pore Strips

Serums
Boots No.7 Protect & Perfect
Estée Lauder Advanced Night Repair
Christian Dior Capture Totale Multi-
Perfection Concentrated Treatment
  Serum
L'Oréal Age Perfect Intensive
Reinforcing Serum
Shiseido Benefiance NutriPerfect Eye
  Serum

MAKEUP

Foundations
Full Coverage
Bobbi Brown Foundation Stick
Becca Foundation Stick
MAC Full Coverage Foundation

Medium to Full Coverage
MAC Studio Sculpt Foundation

Sheer Coverage
MAC Face and Body Foundation

Oil Free/Oil Control
Nars Oil Free Foundation

Illuminating
Chanel Vitalumière Foundation
Giorgio Armani Foundation

Moisturizing
Bobbi Brown Luminous
Moisturizing Foundation

Cream to Powder
MAC Studio Tech Foundation
Shu Uemura Nobara Cream
   Foundation

Powder-Based
MAC Studio Fix

Liquid
RMK Liquid Foundation

Mousse
Lancôme Magie Matte Mousse
Max Factor Miracle Touch
   Foundation
Maybelline Dream Matte Mousse
   Foundation

Tinted Moisturizer
Becca Luminous Skin Colour
Laura Mercier Tinted Moisturizer

For Dark Skins
Armani Fluid Sheer in Golden
   Bronze or Sienna
Bobbi Brown Foundation Stick
Becca Luminous Skin Colour and
   Stick Foundation
Becca Shimmering Skin Perfector
   in Bronze or Topaz
Giorgio Armani Face Fabric
   Second Skin Nude Makeup
MAC Studio Tech Foundation

For Asian/Latin/Indian Skins
Bobbi Brown Foundation Stick
Becca Tinted Moisturizer and
   Stick Foundation
Giorgio Armani Designer Shaping
   Cream Foundation SPF 20
Lancôme Photogenic Lumessence
   Foundation
MAC Mineralize Foundation

Concealer
Bobbi Brown Creamy Concealer
Estée Lauder Smoothing Skin
   Concealer
Laura Mercier Secret Camouflage
Revlon New Complexion Concealer

Blusher
Becca Lip and Cheek Cream
Benefit Posie Tint
MAC Cheek Cream
Maybelline Dream Mousse Blush

Highlighter
MAC Strobe Cream
Yves Saint Laurent Touche Éclat

Contouring
MAC Sculpt & Shape Powder

Powder
Full Coverage
MAC Mineralize Skin Finish Powder
MAC Studio Fix

Sheer Powder
Ben Nye Loose Powder
Shu Uemura Loose Powder

Loose Pigment Powders
Barry M Dazzle Dust
Kryolan Living Color

Eye Primer
Benefit Lemon Aid

Eyeshadow
Bobbi Brown Longwear cream
eyeshadow
Shu Uemura

Eyeliner
MAC Fluidline gel eyeliner

Lips
Lip Primers/Concealers
Benefit Lip Plump
MAC Lip Erase
MAC Prep + Prime Lip

Exfoliators
Hollywood Lip Sweet Sugar Scrub
   and Soothing Day Relief
Rodial Glam Balm

Sheer Colour
Laura Mercier Bare Lips
Benefit Benetint

Matte Colour
MAC Russian Red

Cream Texture
Benefit Lady's Choice

Frost
Revlon Silver City Pink

Opaque
MAC CB96

Gloss
MAC Clear Lipglass

ABOUT AOFM

The Academy of Freelance Makeup is set in the buzzing and exciting surroundings of London's Soho. AOFM has become London's number one makeup school in fashion, editorial, catwalk and bridal makeup – it is the place to learn the skills and gain the experience you need to start your career as a budding makeup artist.

AOFM firmly believes the only way to truly understand how the industry operates is to learn from the people who are working in the business right now. All of their tutors are current working artists, many of them from renowned agencies. This enables them to demonstrate the latest styles and techniques from fashion and catwalk shows and advertising campaigns from all over the world.

With Versace, Armani, Dior and Italian *Vogue* among the names on their client lists, AOFM tutors are some of the most talented in the game. Each tutor has exceptional creative flair in their respective fields, providing students with exposure to a variety of different styles and techniques.

The Academy is one of the only institutes sponsored and supported by a number of famous cosmetic and hair companies. This gives students the opportunity to work with these companies and their products, giving them exposure to a variety of different brands.

AOFM are also proud to offer their students invaluable work experience and jobs within the industry after completing their courses due to their strong relationships and contacts within the industry. Students leave the academy well prepared and with a thorough understanding of the business, giving them an invaluable headstart to their career.

Unique assisting opportunities include prestigious fashion events such as London Fashion Week, where AOFM is a sponsor of many shows (heading up on average 60 shows a year), New York Fashion Week, the *Clothes Show Live* and *Britain's Next Top Model*. Advertorial and editorial shoots within a number of high-profile media channels include British and Italian *Vogue*, MTV and X Factor. The AOFM Pro Team are well-known experts within the industry and are often asked to provide seasonal trends, expert quotes and hints and tips for fashion and beauty brands such as Chloé, Versace and L'Oréal. Celebrity clients include Girls Aloud, the Pussycat Dolls and Giselle.

AOFM is in a league of its own, offering students and makeup wannabes all the advantages of learning from top working makeup artists. They have built a unrivalled reputation in training professional artists and their world-renowned creative Pro Team travel all over the globe demonstrating their skills.

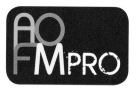

Academy of Freelance Makeup
63 Dean Street
Soho, London W1D 4QG
Tel: 020 7434 4488
www.aofmakeup.com
email info@aofmakeup.com

ACKNOWLEDGMENTS

We would like to say a special thank you to the following model agencies and PR for all their support:

Robert Hannan at Next Models, Teoh Gold at Nevs, Kai at FM Agency, Maxine Henshilwood at Oxygen, Trix Stephenson at First Model Management, Khalid El Awad and James Clark at IMG Models, Russell and Charlie at M&P Model Management.

Aude at Christian Dior, Christina Aristodemou and Jo Scicluna at MAC Artist Relations, Lisa Nash and Helen at Shu Uemura, Jenna at Becca, Claire and Dafna at Bobbi Brown, Samantha at KMS, Caroline Young at St Tropez, Raj Kaur and the team at Lancôme, Jess at Purple PR, Clair at Benefit Cosmetics, Alison and the marketing team at Dermalogica, Nicky at Redken, the team at Dowal Walker PR for all their support, Jane at Illamasqua, Mary at Jessica Nails, Zoe at Chanel, Candice at Balcony Jump management, the team at Blow PR, Sophie Stanbury and the team at Swarovski, Chris Manoe and the team at International Collective, Mark Whittel at No. 5 Cavendish for the use of location and hospitality. And finally a special thanks to Jaon Mallett and Ioannis Pagonis.,

AFTERWORD

"After years of writing about beauty, directing beauty and fashion shoots and working with so many talented makeup artists, I decided I wanted to put my pen down, pick up my blusher brush and get a little more hands on with makeup. This is what led me to the Academy of Freelance Makeup to train as a makeup artist. That was a few years ago, and today I have my pen back in my hand to scribble what I hope have been some helpful notes and corrections to this fabulous book, and to write these final words.

Makeup artists are a thing of wonder to me. Over the years, I have watched them transform models, real women and celebrities into works of art. It always has – and always will – amaze me how beauty products can hold such power. They have the ability to instantly boost confidence, hide all manner of sins, highlight beautiful features and be the tools to create something so special that it can take your breath away.

This book shows how, with creative thinking, ability and sheer determination, you can become a makeup artist and when the imagination is set free, beauty can be created from beauty.

So, although I have my pen back in one hand, I will always have my blusher brush in the other."

Sarah-Jane Corfield-Smith,
Lifestyle Journalist

INDEX

Figures in italics indicate captions.

{overleaf}
Photographer: Camille Sanson
Makeup: Lan Nguyen using MAC and Swarovski. Jewellery by Louis Mariette

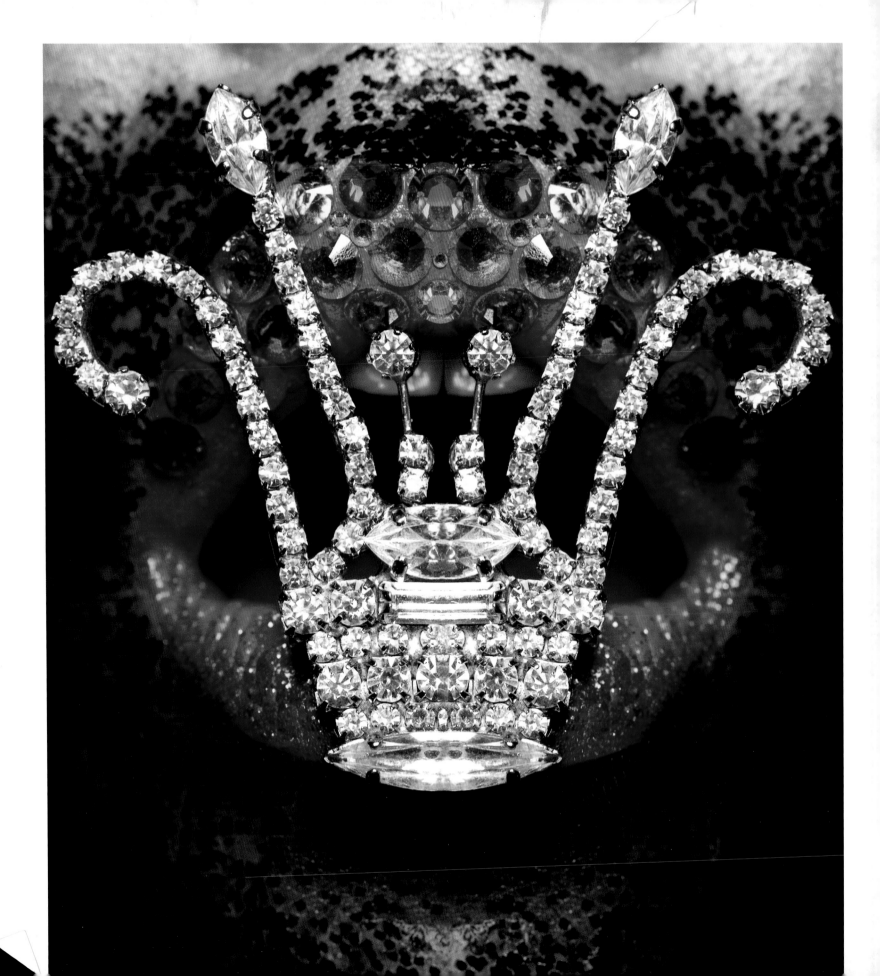